"Deborah Cohen and Robert Gelfand, M.D., have written a very thoughtful, warm and complete guidebook for women diagnosed with breast cancer. This book has a lovely but realistic tone and will be helpful for patients, their families and friends. I highly recommend it."

—Alison Estabrook, M.D., F.A.C.S.
Chief of Breast Surgery,
St. Luke's Roosevelt Hospital
Professor of Clinical Surgery,
Columbia University

"Just Get Me Through This! will help all women facing breast cancer to muster the strength and summon the courage needed to put one foot in front of the other and walk step-by-step through breast cancer, one day and one decision at a time—all with a bit of humor and perspective from someone who's been there."

—Andrea Martin
Founder and Executive Director
The Breast Cancer Fund

"It is not often that I find myself praising a 'self-help' book for patients with breast cancer, since so many of them, frankly, are repetitive and condescending to the reader. *Just Get Me Through This!* is certainly the exception. The authors—a woman who's been there and an oncologist with extensive experience—take you by the hand and expertly guide you through the day-ins and day-outs of managing everything about your breast cancer. This is not only a practical coping guide, but also offers a unique perspective on each decision associated with surgery and treatment."

—Pablo J. Cagnoni, M.D.
Assistant Professor of Medicine
University of Colorado Bone
Marrow Transplant Program
University of Colorado Cancer Center

JUST GET ME THROUGH THIS!

A Practical Guide To Coping With Breast Cancer

Newly Revised and Updated

Deborah A. Cohen and

Robert M. Gelfand, M.D.,
with Eugene J. Nowak, M.D.
and Faith A. Menken, M.D.

KENSINGTON BOOKS
www.kensingtonbooks.com

The authors and publisher assert that all information contained herein is accurate to the best of their knowledge. It is based not only on the authors' personal experiences, but also on anecdotal research from interviews with both medical professionals and breast cancer survivors. However, in no case should any information be interpreted or construed as clinical medical advice, and under no circumstances can the authors or any contributors be held liable for the outcome or result of any action taken based upon advice or information contained in this book. If medical advice is required, the services of a competent professional should be sought.

KENSINGTON BOOKS are published by

Kensington Publishing Corp.
119 W. 40th Street
New York, NY 10018

All Kensington titles, imprints, and distributed lines are available at special quantity discounts for bulk purchases for sales promotion, premiums, fund-raising, educational, or institutional use.

Special book excerpts or customized printings can also be created to fit specific needs. For details, write or phone the office of the Kensington Special Sales Manager: Kensington Publishing Corp., 119 West 40th Street, New York, NY 10018. Attn. Special Sales Department. Phone: 1-800-221-2647.

Kensington and the K logo Reg. U.S. Pat. & TM Off.

ISBN-13: 978-0-7582-6953-9
ISBN-10: 0-7582-6953-6

First Printing: May 2000
First Revised Printing: September 2003
Second Revised Printing: September 2011
20 19 18 17 16 15 14 13 12 11 10 9 8 7 6 5 4

Printed in the United States of America

CONTENTS

DEDICATION

This book is especially dedicated to:

- My mother, Myrna, whose own life-debilitating illness has brought new meaning to the word *courage*.
- My father, Don, who is a pillar of stability, even when his world is crumbling around him.
- My brother, Dan, who helped me maintain my sanity and perspective in times of seeming chaos.
- My aunt, Elaine, who taught me what nurturing and support are really all about.
- My "Vermont mom," Ginny, who stepped in at just the right critical moments.
- All the incredible friends that have been there for me, both old and new, whom I am so blessed to have in my life. You know who you are and I love you all. . . .

I would also like to recognize several other individuals without whose efforts and understanding this book would never have become a reality:

- My "shadow" agent, Helen, who saw the jewel in the glimmer of an idea, and pushed me to make it happen.
- My current boss, Susan, who graciously and patiently accommodated my work schedule around her belief in this project.

- My editorial advisor, John, whom I revere for his journalistic brilliance and editorial rigor.
- My editor, Tracy Bernstein, who humored me past obstacles in the road to completion.
- And last, but far from least, my coauthor, Rob, who kept me on course when I began to stray, and calm in the midst of the storm, in more ways than one.

I feel honored and privileged to have had such a talented group of individuals providing such support, encouragement, and friendship throughout this endeavor.

Deborah Cohen

This book is dedicated to:

- My beautiful wife, Jody, and our wonderful girls, Madeline, Erica, and Jessica.
- My mentors and friends, to whom I owe more than I can ever repay—Anne, Arnie, Mort, and Rob.
- Deborah, who will always be an inspiration to me.

Robert Gelfand

A NOTE FROM THE AUTHORS

This book is intended specifically for women with early-stage breast cancer. Yes, "cancer" is a terrifying word that immediately conjures up visions of mortality and unfulfilled dreams. Yet with the miracles of the modern medical world today, early-stage breast cancer is, for the most part, a treatable, manageable disease. It *will*, as everyone will tell you, profoundly change you and your attitude toward life—life, not death. It will often be on your mind, just like any other chronic disease. Yet it need *not* diminish the quality of your long and healthy life. You *will* grow old, hopefully. And you probably will see the cure in your lifetime. We hope the advice and wisdom contained herein is helpful, insightful, and uplifting.

ACKNOWLEDGMENTS

We would like to gratefully acknowledge all those medical experts, other professionals, and survivors who graciously donated their time and insights. Your perspectives were invaluable in providing us with both factually correct information and a sound basis for forming the opinions expressed throughout the book on how to address a multitude of experiences and situations.

Overall Perspective: Andrea Martin, Executive Director, The Breast Cancer Fund, San Francisco.

Surgery: Eugene J. Nowak, M.D., New York Hospital/Cornell Medical Center, New York.

Medical Oncology: Larry Norton, M.D., Chief of Solid Tumor Medicine, Memorial Sloan-Kettering Cancer Center, New York; Greg Berk, M.D., New York Hospital/Cornell Medical Center, New York.

Radiation Oncology: Beryl McCormick, M.D., Department of Radiation Oncology, Memorial Sloan-Kettering Cancer Center, New York; Alison Grann, M.D., Department of Radiation Oncology, Memorial Sloan-Kettering Cancer Center, New York; Alfred Rosenbaum, M.D., Assistant Clinical Professor of Radiology, Mt. Sinai School of Medicine, New York.

Psychooncology: David Payne, Ph.D., Psychologist, Department of Psychiatry and Behavioral Sciences, Memorial Sloan-Kettering Cancer Center, New York.

Dentistry: Thomas J. Magnani, D.D.S., New York.

Alopecia/Hair Loss: Gwen Bourhis, Barry Hendrickson's Bitz-n-Pieces Salon, New York.

Prostheses: Marion Kieves and Carol Art Keane, Underneath It All, New York.

Dermatology: David E. Cohen, M.D., M.P.H., New York University Medical Center, New York.

Mammography: Danielle Carbone, imaging systems specialist.

Gynecology: Charles J. Bacall, M.D., Attending Obstetrician-Gynecologist, Mt. Sinai Hospital, New York, Private Practice.

Alternative Medicine: Raymond Chang, M.D., Meridian Medical Group, New York.

Nutrition: Courtney Gravenese, M.S., RD, Clinical Research Dietician, Memorial Sloan-Kettering Cancer, New York; Betty Reiser, Director, SHARE: Self Help for Women with Breast or Ovarian Cancer, New York.

Financial, Legal, Employment, Insurance: S. Susan Slavin, Esq., Slavin Law Firm, Jericho, New York; Kelly A. Martz, President, Healthcare Administration Management Corp., Montebello, New York; Katherine Tsougranis, Human Resources, Pricewaterhouse-Coopers, New York.

Editorial: John Thackray, Editorial Advisor, New York; Judy Baron, Copyediting, Chicago; Nancy Cesari, President, NameLogic, Dallas.

Women Survivors: And a heartfelt expression of gratitude to the many truly amazing women I spoke with and interviewed, both formally and informally, especially Roberta F., Sara H., Kim O., Claudia S., Carolyn O., Kate M., Mary C., and Ellen G.. Your courage, spirit, perseverance, and candor should be an inspiration to everyone, and your advice and wisdom of particular help to all women yet to embark on their own unique breast cancer journey.

FOREWORD
BY DR. GELFAND

Over the past decade there has been a growing movement in the practice of medicine—patient advocacy. Patients are increasingly taking charge of their own health and taking steps to be well informed and active in decisions about their own bodies. The passive patient with a "whatever-you-say-Doc" attitude is becoming the exception rather than the norm. However, in the case of a serious, complex illness like breast cancer, the proactive patient may end up confused, overwhelmed with information, and excessively anxious. The saying that "a little knowledge is dangerous" is apt for these situations. The acquisition of great amounts of technical information by breast cancer patients without medical training—from books or extensive exploring on the Internet—frequently ends up aggravating the anxiety. A lot of the questions that I get asked by breast cancer patients reflect their earnest attempts at self-education but also their minimal understanding of the complexity of the underlying issues, or knowledge of how the information should be organized and utilized.

Women with breast cancer, and their family and friends, most of all need a balanced approach to this illness. They need a basic road map to help them deal with the up-and-down journey from diagnosis into the world of the "patient" and back to the world of "normalcy"—a map that outlines the major phases of the process, offers guidance and insights along the way, and presents basic technical information in simple, understandable language. *Just Get Me Through This!* strives for balance through the collaboration of a seasoned professional and an intelligent patient. The result is neither a technical manual to breast cancer, nor a personal biography of overcoming breast cancer. Rather we have blended the perspectives of doctor and patient—enhanced by extensive conversations with other medical professionals, patients, and survivors—to offer readers a well-rounded, straight-from-the-shoulder view of the illness and of appropriate responses. We do not aim to be the only source of information and insight that you will need. We simply offer a foundation on which to build trusting, open dialogue not only with your health care team (e.g., surgeons, oncologists, nurses), but with family, friends, and even coworkers.

One of the most important and least written about aspects of breast cancer is the degree to which the diagnosis alters one's life experience. By and large doctors do not prepare patients for more than the technical aspects of treatment. For example, doctors will go to great lengths to explain the powers of today's highly effective antinausea drugs, but they will rarely help a patient manage the inevitable emotional traumas, anxieties, and practical difficulties of chemotherapy. Few surgeons will discuss the fact that a spouse or significant other might have difficulty coping with the results of a mastectomy or other bodily changes, and recommend ways to improve communication to work through such tough relationship issues. And who warns a patient of the possible coldness and even disappearance of old friends who are terrified by her cancer diagnosis because of their own issues with mortality?

Yes, it is wonderful and comforting to learn from your doctor that chemotherapy and all the other conventional medical treatments available today are typically well tolerated as long as the symptoms are managed well, and that by and large most women go on to live normal lives in the aftermath of cancer. Yet it is the nonmedical facets, the gestalt of the whole breast cancer experience, that most of the 200,000 women a year diagnosed with breast cancer are unprepared for. We have written *Just Get Me Through This!* to address that need. It is our hope that when you have turned the last page, you will find the knowledge empowering, the insight balanced from both the human and treatment perspectives, and the empathy offered by the authors comforting.

Robert M. Gelfand, M.D.
Clinical Assistant Professor of Medicine
Weill Medical College of Cornell University

FOREWORD
BY DR. MENKEN AND DR. NOWAK

We are honored to have been asked to contribute to this newest printing of this very special book. In rereading the prior edition, written just a few years ago, we were sharply reminded of the progress we have made in the surgical management of patients with breast cancer. Treatments that were just a short time ago experimental, controversial, or not even conceived of yet have now become routine. As such, we hope that our input as surgeons will be a valuable edition to Dr. Gelfand's medical input in helping patients to understand their treatment options better, and to navigate this sometimes daunting process.

As physicians, we do our best to educate, guide, and reassure our patients. The surgeon is most often the first breast "expert" the patient meets. His or her empathy, understanding, and approachability are of paramount importance. We often set the tone for the patient's experience. Our ability to communicate is every bit as important as our surgical skills.

Nothing, however, can be as reassuring as hearing from someone who has made it through the journey. For this reason, we are proud to be a part of what must be considered Debbie Cohen's labor of love.

Faith A. Menken, M.D.

Eugene J. Nowak, M.D.

INTRODUCTION

I want to talk to you for a moment about Fudgsicles.

"Fudgsicles? Are you crazy? I have a life-threatening disease and you want to talk to me about Fudgsicles?!?! Can't you just help me get through this?"

Yes, believe it or not, I do want to talk about Fudgsicles, as they actually may be very important in helping you get through the next six to nine months of your life. Here's why.

When I was recovering from my initial surgery, I was bombarded with advice from friends and family about books to read on cancer treatments, in order to be prepared to talk with surgeons, oncologists, and other specialists about the best course of treatment for my disease. This is the new world of health care, and I am the perfect model of the "patient activist." I wanted to be involved in a true partnership with the doctors to make decisions about my own body and my own life. I was not going to sit there and simply be told what to do. Yet I found it wasn't all that easy.

When I visited my local bookstore to begin my process of becoming an informed patient, I almost passed out in the aisleway—from terror, not from my illness. The vast majority of books were harsh, clinical reference materials, written solely by doctors, chock-full of terrifying mortality statistics. They talked about how sick I was going to get, either from the disease or from the treatments to eradicate the disease, not how to manage the treatments and get well. The remainder were heroic biographies by cancer patients themselves—some survivors, some not—about their own courageous battles. No thanks, I have my own battle to contend with right here at home. I don't need to read about anyone else's right now.

So, I threw away all those books, and started talking to people—doctors, nurses, survivors, whoever would talk to me—and it was amazing what I learned, what similar, consistent information started coming back to me regardless of the source. A flagship example? Before I went for my first chemotherapy treatment, I had three different people—one oncologist, one chemotherapy nurse, and one of the women in my support group who had been through the same treatment regimen—tell me that during the ten to fifteen minutes that the drug Adriamycin is being administered to me, I should suck on ice chips, Popsicles, or something cold. Why? Because one of the potential side effects of that particular drug is mouth and gum sores. But for some reason, sucking on something cold minimizes or even eradicates mouth sores.

Now, where was *that* book, the book that contained all of that nitty-gritty, practical advice that would just get me through the next six months—the operating guide, the instruction manual, the *"how to's"* of breast cancer? It didn't exist. So, I started an information-gathering process, which I've presented here in a package called a book. It contains all those practical "tidbits" of advice gathered from every conceivable source—from breast surgeons, medical and radiation oncologists, and nurses at some of the world's leading cancer centers; from health care consultants and medical literature; from nutritionists, hairdressers, dentists, and other personal-care professionals; from fellow patients and support groups; and even from plain old books. I personally sifted, sorted, and tested their advice, insights, anecdotes, and even their wives' tales, then added my own perspective.

So now the book exists, and you are reading it. We don't know if or why sucking on Popsicles prevents mouth sores—it may be that just as the cold restricts blood flow, it restricts chemotherapy flow to the area—but it sure helps many, many women. And wouldn't it make those potentially unpleasant, dark, scary moments just a bit more tolerable? I actually prefer Fudgsicles, please, but I was willing to do whatever it took to get me through treatment. But wait. There's more than that to our discussion of Fudgsicles. This book is not only about advice, but about attitude as well. Fudgsicles bring us back to childhood, back to those carefree, breezy summer evenings when the highlight was sitting on the front porch with our best friend and guessing what time the ice cream man would turn the corner onto our street, ringing his bell and bringing a smile to the faces of all who awaited him. This book is also about rediscovering those slower, simpler moments of life, about recouping that positive attitude from childhood that each day promises something special and something new to be discovered, if only we take a minute to open our eyes and look.

Breast cancer is an eye-opening, life-affirming experience. You may think it won't change your life, that you're tough, that you can just keep on going and functioning in the life-is-normal-as-possible mode. But you can't. As everyone tells you, and as you won't believe, it will change your life in many ways:

- You will look at life in a whole new way, as something you are lucky to be experiencing.
- You will appreciate every day, just because it is there and has been given to you to enjoy.
- You won't take your health for granted, and will take better care of your mind and your body, making *yourself* a priority (rather than your family, friends, job, or other distractions).
- You will be calmer . . . the little things won't seem to bother you as much.
- You won't worry about tomorrow as much, but live for today.
- You will draw nearer to the people who bring meaning and fulfillment to your life, and get rid of those who don't (crises have an amazing way of revealing someone's true character).
- You will gain extreme clarity . . . about exactly who you are and what you want from your life.

For many women I encountered, this experience gave them the courage to take action regarding major decisions in their lives that they had been postponing or evading—getting out of bad relationships even though they might have been comfortable, leaving dead-end jobs, reevaluating relationships with estranged family members. After all, once you've been through breast cancer, nothing else seems quite as ominous or overwhelming.

Yes, there's no going back. Life will now always be divided into "before B.C." and "after B.C." As I sat in my gynecologist's office, discussing what it meant that my lab tests were returned showing "malignant" cells, he said, "You won't believe it now, but good things will come out of this." Yeah, right! Now, many months and many tears later, slowly but surely, I am starting to believe him.

Above all, this book is about optimism. It is about how to look for those good things that will arise out of this experience, about focusing on long-term survival and lifetime plans, and about finding some humor and maintaining a sense of sanity in the midst of seeming chaos. The six-to-twelve-month experience of diagnosis, surgery, and treatment can seem interminably long, like a never-ending marathon, a gauntlet of professionals pushing, poking, and invading your body, followed by a proliferation of advice upon which no two professionals seem to agree. But you will get through it, and here, in the pages that follow, is your step-by-step guide to help you through the chaos, catastrophe, and turmoil of the entire breast cancer experience.

The book is organized into four sections of chronological progression, from that disbelieving moment of diagnosis to that anticlimactic, ever-elusive "finish" to the treatment, and that strange transition period back to real life. We will cover:

- The Diagnosis—*Managing the News* that you have cancer, including comprehending it yourself, and determining how and when to communicate it to the broader world; and *Swinging into Action,* which provides perspectives on gathering the information you need to make informed decisions, establishing your emotional support and coping mechanisms, and building the best health care team you can find to assist you in your journey.
- Surgery—*Deciding on Surgery* offers an explanation and factors to determine which surgical alternatives might be appropriate for you; *Undergoing Surgery* provides an overview of the surgical experience and what to expect from the hospital visit; and *Recovering from Surgery* sets forth what you can expect from your body, emotions, and the actual surgical results.

- Treatment—*Deciphering Treatment Alternatives* discusses the plethora of choices available, how they work, and why your health care team might recommend various options for you; *Managing Treatments: Chemotherapy and Radiation* delineates all the practical advice you need for getting through both the process of treatment and its impact on your life, as well as managing any physical side effects and balancing demands of the workplace.
- Getting Back to Life—*Ending Treatment* explores the often surprising issues you may face in your transition back to your "normal" life (although you will never quite be able to go back to where you came from); *Maintaining a Healthy Lifestyle* offers suggestions on how nutrition and the world of alternative medicine can optimize your strength and well-being.

Sprinkled throughout the text are portions written by Dr. Robert M. Gelfand entitled "A Note from the Doctor," which explain some of the more clinical technical aspects of managing breast cancer. And at the end of each section, you'll even find some "Rules of the Road" directed to family, friends, and others who will accompany you on your journey through breast cancer.

So before we get into the guts of this book, you're probably wondering just who I am and why I am writing this book. What makes me the expert? Unfortunately for us both, I may be just like you. Nothing made me the expert until one day without any warning this ominous disease called breast cancer reared its ugly head and slapped me in the face. No family history, no other health issues, nothing. I'm just a fairly normal person with a normal life, who could be your friend, coworker, next-door neighbor, wife, sister, or daughter.

All in all, my life up to now has been good. No, it hasn't been perfect, but in retrospect, it's been pretty terrific, now that it's been threatened to be taken away from me. I've been blessed with a close family, incredible friends, a never-ending array of interesting professional challenges and coworkers, and a wide variety of athletic, intellectual, and social interests and activities. I've seen a lot of the world and learned to appreciate what I have, and to be content to know that there will always be things that I might never have.

But perhaps most important to you, my diagnosis helped me realize that, if caught in its early stages, breast cancer is not a catastrophic disease, but merely a potentially catastrophic situation. My expertise comes from experience, from being able to offer real-world, in-the-trenches, been-there guidance on how to manage your way through—and thereby avert—physical, emotional, and even financial catastrophe.

And finally, just to be safe, I recruited Dr. Robert M. Gelfand, an oncologist whom I encountered when I visited him for a second opinion. After he spent more than two hours with me, objectively, but compassionately and patiently, answering each and every one of my questions—no question was too dumb to ask—I was convinced he was to be my co-author. He generously agreed to provide expertise regarding the more technical aspects of the book, and to ensure that nothing I discuss or suggest is harmful or improper.

In this newly updated edition, we have added the input of two esteemed breast surgeons: Drs. Faith Menken and Eugene Nowak. As the care of breast cancer patients has evolved both medically and surgically, input from experienced surgeons has surfaced as a clear need. Hopefully, you will find this addition to be of great value.

So, enter breast cancer.

PART I

THE DIAGNOSIS

CHAPTER 1
Managing the News

There is no good way to receive the news that's the single fear beyond your worst dreams—that you have cancer. No, not somebody else, but you. This chapter will cover a few ways to handle this nightmare over the first few days, in terms of:

- *Comprehending* the news yourself, and communicating it to those few people who need to know as soon as possible, both for your sake, if only to be able to vocalize it, and theirs.
- *Reacting* to the news, and a few ideas for giving yourself a helpful perspective on the situation.
- *Spreading* the news, and determining how broadly and by what means to expose yourself to the "outside" world.

COMPREHENDING AND COMMUNICATING THE NEWS: AN UNEXPECTED TIDAL WAVE

Malignant Cells: Are Those the Good Ones or the Bad Ones?

It's 4 P.M. on a Thursday afternoon, and I'm waiting for a meeting to begin in my office. The phone rings and I decide to answer it while I await my guest. I had been to see a "breast specialist" forty-eight hours earlier for a biopsy on a lump I had found on the side of my breast, but to be honest, I hadn't thought twice about it since. He had reassured me, "It's probably nothing. With women your age, most likely—80 percent chance—it's just a fibrous knot." I had no family history, knew nobody who had breast or any other cancer in my age group, so I had just put it out of my mind.

No more; actually, never again. When I answered the phone, he got straight to the point. "Hello, this is Gene Nowak. I'm sorry to tell you this, but the lab tests showed some malignant cells in your biopsy, which will require treatment." *Malignant?* Are malignant cells the good ones or the bad ones? I could tell by the tone of his voice that malignancies didn't exactly bring you the winnings of a lottery ticket, but what did he mean? Did he mean *cancer?* I had only known two people with cancer, and they were older relatives of mine, my grandfather and my uncle, more than ten years ago each. I knew that "lumps," tumors, or cysts—whatever you call them—were classified as either malignant or benign, but I didn't know which was okay and which meant cancer. It just wasn't on my radar screen. It was irrelevant to my young, healthy, active life. *Treatment?* What does *that* mean? Is it surgery? Or does it mean lots of other medical "procedures" that are terrifying, so the doctors don't tell you the potentially far-reaching implications of them now, because you have enough to swallow today? My head was spinning.

So, I queried, "Dr. Nowak, does this mean I have *c-c-c-c-cancer?*" And he responded, "Yes, unfortunately it does. Why don't you come see me tomorrow morning when I have some time to sit with you and thoroughly discuss your alternatives." Tomorrow morning? Can I wait until then? Will I still be alive!? I was in shock. I managed to get out, "Okay. What time?" Then I put the phone down. Now the entire room was spinning. I was shaking and my heart dropped to my stomach. I called my mother. "Mom, the biopsy is back and it shows some malignant cells." "What???" she responded. "Mother, I have *breast cancer,*" I replied, deliberately pronouncing each word. And as I hung up the phone on her because those were the only words I could muster, my meeting guest was standing at my office door. I looked up and said, "I have to cancel our meeting and go home. My doctor just told me I have *cancer.*" And I picked up my coat to leave. Yes, malignant cells are the bad ones. And there, I had even said the "c" word three times. As I left the office, I knew that somehow my life had changed forever, but I was not yet quite sure how. All I knew was that I felt as if I had been smacked in the face by a tidal wave. Somehow, I would have to pick myself up and put myself back together again.

A NOTE FROM THE ONCOLOGIST

℞ **What's Malignant, What's Benign, and What's Metastatic? Cell Growth Formation 101**

Every cell in your body has a specific function. Brain cells transport neurological messages, stomach cells help digest and absorb food, and breast duct cells make milk. Occasionally, however, a change in the chromosome pattern in the DNA of a cell occurs—a "mutation." This can be caused by an inherited defect, external factors such as radiation or environmental toxins, or a combination of the two. Usually, a mutation has no effect at all on the cell—it continues to do its job as "programmed." Sometimes, the mutation is lethal to the cell, so the cell just dies and is washed out of your body (no big deal, we make billions of new cells every day).

Less often, the mutation leads to the transformation of the cell in such a way that it no longer performs its function (e.g., producing milk, telling your hand to move, absorbing your lunch), but rather reprograms itself to simply replicate or "clone" itself. A group of these cells is a tumor. A "benign" tumor does not invade or damage other parts of the body, while a "malignant" tumor will be fueled by and destroy surrounding tissue. In sum, a malignant breast tumor is composed of breast cells that have replicated themselves out of control, overtaking and destroying healthy cells and tissue in their wake.

If you are reading this book as someone with "early-stage" cancer, you are lucky that most likely, all the cancerous cells have remained grouped together in the original tumor site in the breast—that is, your cancer has remained "local." Survival rates are very high for localized, early-stage cancer, and often you are "cured" by surgery alone. All the additional treatment you may undergo is "preventative" or "adjuvant," just extra "insurance" in case microscopic cancerous cells have broken away from your tumor and moved to other parts of your body. When original "clonal" cells migrate from the breast organ to another place in your body and begin forming tumors, that is called a "metastasis." When you hear of cancer "metastasizing," it means that the cancer has spread to other organs—in the case of breast cancer, most commonly the lungs, bones, or liver—and is invading the healthy tissue of those organs.

There Are Many Roads Leading to "Suspicious."

If you're reading this book, unfortunately you may have realized that there are many roads which can lead your doctor to mutter something about "suspicious _____" (fill in the blank). It could be several alternatives: a "lump" you found yourself, either intentionally or accidentally; a "thickening" that your doctor found upon examination; or a mammogram where something caught the doctor's attention. Whatever the pathway there, the next step is typically a biopsy. You must understand the role of the biopsy, and what information you can glean from it before considering your surgical options, if that is the appropriate route. Remember, early-stage cancer is very treatable, with extremely high survival rates. In a strange sort of way, think of yourself as lucky that your doctor was suspicious. It may have saved your life.

A NOTE FROM THE SURGEONS

R̸   *A Biopsy Is a Biopsy . . . or Is It?*

For those of you just beginning the breast cancer journey, you need to be clear about exactly what a biopsy can and can not tell you. While there are variations on each, there are essentially four types of biopsies, which are increasingly invasive, but also increasingly exacting in terms of diagnosis. However, other than a complete surgical biopsy which removes the entire mass, biopsy results are not 100% definitive. Biopsy types are:

1. ***Fine needle aspiration (FNA).*** Conducted in the surgeon's office, this involves inserting a needle into a mass that can be felt and removing representative cells. This is not felt to be a definitive diagnosis, but is still fairly accurate.
2. ***Core biopsy.*** Conducted in the radiologist's office, this uses a sonogram to identify the mass and then a wide bore needle to remove a core of tissue. Definitive surgical decisions can be made on the basis of a core biopsy diagnosis because it provides a bigger sample than FNA.
3. ***Stereotactic core biopsy.*** Conducted in the radiologist's office, this uses a mammogram to detect calcifications or architectural distortions that are not able to be felt. This also takes a core of tissue and uses a special table placing the patient facedown. Definitive surgical decisions can be made on the basis of a stereotactic core biopsy.
4. ***Excisional (open) biopsy.*** Conducted in the operating room using local anesthesia and intravenous sedation, this involves removal of a mass or calcifications that are not technically amenable to either core biopsy or stereotactic biopsy (deep or close to the chest wall, directly behind the nipple, or in patients who cannot be positioned for stereotactic biopsy due to arthritis or other illness).

Regardless of which type of biopsy you had, if there is any debate about the interpretation of the results, consider going to a more extensive procedure. A little sacrifice now of time, pain, and even tissue may save you a lot later.

Getting Your Lab Report . . . like Remembering Where You Were When JFK Was Shot.

Just accept that you will never forget the moment your doctor received the results of your lab test, and had to break the news to you. Just as every American adult has a vivid snapshot branded in their memory of exactly where they were and what they were doing when they heard the news that John F. Kennedy was shot, so will you have an indelible imprint of where you were and how you were told that you have cancer. Just as JFK's assassination became a significant moment in American history, your news will become a part of your heritage, your strength, who you are. No matter how much you want to rewind the clock and erase it, you can't. Cancer is now part of your history.

A Dose of Quiet Time Is the Best Medicine for the Ordeal Ahead.

No matter what your point of origin, be it your family physician, your gynecologist, a breast specialist, or even a dermatologist, if you are reading this book, all roads have led you to this shocking crossroads. Like me, you now have cancer as a relevant term in your life—for the rest of it! However, as you will see throughout this book, this news is not a destination, or an end, but the beginning of a new journey—a journey that will redefine who you are and what you want from life, a journey that has obstacles, but also high points, and a journey that many others will share with you and help you endure. However, in the immediate aftermath of receiving your diagnosis, allow yourself some moments alone to just sit and let it sink in as much as it can. Maybe you already have by the time you're reading this. But if you haven't, get away to places that make you feel good. If you like art, go to a gallery or museum. If you like the outdoors, go for a hike or walk in the nearest park. Don't necessarily *do* anything yet. Look at the surroundings you've chosen, and realize how little you actually see on a daily basis, until news like this makes you wake up to the details of the world around you. Realize how lucky you are just to be sitting there. These moments alone will allow you to get your head clear enough to understand what is happening to you, determine who you need to share your news with, in what order, how, and when. And if you haven't already, use some of this time to make lists of all the questions you want to ask your doctor and all the people who can possibly help you and might know something about your new disease.

A Three-Phase Plan for Letting the News Sink in.

The news that you have breast cancer cannot be comprehended in a single dose. It's something that may happen in phases over several days—easing into your consciousness, and understanding that, "Yes, they are talking about me." And while you will come to understand that fact, it will actually take months, perhaps years, to fully comprehend the implications of that little piece of news. So, after that initial life-changing phone call from your doctor, here's a simple three-phase plan that I used to handle myself in the transition from healthy person to breast cancer patient (at least temporarily):

Phase 1. Building Your Inner Circle: A State of Shock as the Means to Maintaining Composure.

First, determine who in your immediate world needs to know about this right away, if only to keep you from crumbling emotionally. Your list might include traditional family members such as your spouse/significant other, children, siblings and parents. But think carefully. Your traditional family may not be as much support as you need, for any number of reasons—they won't handle the news well themselves, they are preoccupied with illnesses or life challenges of their own, they are geographically distant, etc. Perhaps there are a few other people who should be included in this "inner circle" of support, people who you know will provide that rock-solid pillar of emotional stability that you'll need for the next several months. Consider them surrogate family. Choose about four or five people. See them in person, if possible, so they can see you, touch you, and know that you are the same person. Otherwise call them. But regardless of how you contact them, please soften the shock a bit by prefacing your news with a comment like, "I have something to tell you, but please hear this first . . . I will be fine . . ."

Despite vocalizing your news, you might still be in shock and not believe this is happening to you. Like me, you might not have even shed one tear yet. That's okay, you're numb. (Or maybe you have. And that's okay too.) Even as I tried to sleep that first night, I didn't cry. But I did lie awake all night, shivering so uncontrollably that my teeth chattered, out of terror, fear, and uncertainty of what lay ahead. . . .

Phase 2. First Cry, See Your Doctor . . . Then Do Something Spectacular.

As the numbness wears off and reality sets in, you might start to cry, and have moments when you just can't stop. That is absolutely normal. After a while, you'll feel the need to pull yourself together. I found that two things helped put a stop to my crying. First, have the consultation with your doctor to identify all the issues you need to address, and determine the options you have to remove the cancer. Bring someone from your "inner circle" with you to take notes on what the doctor recommends. In your state of mind, you might be listening, but you won't hear, let alone comprehend, everything.

By just knowing that there are a lot of options for you to eradicate this cancer from your body and your life, you will feel much better. The doctor might discuss lumpectomy versus mastectomy, radiation, chemotherapy, even hormone therapy. Yes, it is terrifying, but it also can provide a strange sense of calm. Although I had never been in a hospital in my entire life—except the day I was born—I felt great relief knowing that soon I would have surgery to get the cancer out of me. In fact, the surgery was scheduled for a few weeks later, but I was so panicked that the cancer was multiplying exponentially by the minute that I asked the doctor to move the surgery date sooner. Eight days later, I had a lumpectomy and axillary lymph node dissection. (See the discussion in Chapter 3, "Deciding on Surgery.")

The second approach is to do something that absorbs all of your concentration. After a doctor's visit that airs all the issues you'll have to address over the next several months, do something spectacular, something completely out of the ordinary of your daily routine. Do something that takes your full attention, that raises others' expectations of you, that has absolutely nothing to do with your current trauma. In my case, I had to go to work and, in fact, had scheduled interviews with senior executives for a book project we were deep in the midst of. So I walked out of the doctor's office, wiped my tears dry yet one more time, and pulled out the company's annual report on the way to their offices. After all, I needed to know what the company did before I could intelligently interview! I had to be "on" and could not re-schedule. So, with eyes as pink as the magenta suit I was wearing that day, I conducted my interviews, just as if life were "normal."

If you are fortunate enough not to have to go to work, then do something that will make you smile, but make sure you are around other people to distract you. Take your children to an amusement park. Have an extra-long exercise session at your gym to make yourself feel really good. Work on any community activities you might be involved in that make you feel good about helping others less fortunate than you. Just don't think about yourself for the time being.

Phase 3. Expand Your Inner Circle: Break the News, Be Surprised.

By the time you move into the third phase, you may be composed enough to start breaking your news to a wider circle of people. While you might worry that telling others will make you feel like a leper, believe it or not, it will make you feel better. I decided to expand my initial inner circle by calling my six closest friends in the world, regardless of where they lived, to tell them the news, but also tell them that I was going to really need them to be there for me during the coming months. Guess what? Of this small sampling of women, women whom I thought I knew so well, each had an acquaintance or coworker who had been through breast cancer and was completely fine! My own spontaneous sample had a survival rate of 100 percent! They even told inspirational stories of women who had gone on to marry, have children, start new careers, etc. This was great! Not only did I no longer feel all alone in the world, but I learned very early that plenty of women *do* get through this experience (hence, my title), and that my friends would be there to help me.

Determine who else you might want to tell your news personally rather than having them hear indirectly by word-of-mouth. However, make sure that these are people who will be supportive, optimistic, and hopeful. Let them know that, as part of your inner circle, they will be counted on to play several roles for you over the coming months. (See page 3, "Communicating the News.") You don't need to pick anyone else up off the floor right now.

It's Only Two Easy Syllables, but It Might Take Some Time to Be Able to Say the "C" Word.

The word *cancer* is everywhere in our society. On a nearly daily basis, the news bombards us. We are informed of some new medical treatment for some type of cancer, made aware of some fundraising effort for cancer research, or reminded of yet someone else who has been diagnosed or passed away from cancer. But when the word becomes personally attached to your own individual identity, it becomes much more difficult to verbalize. It may take you several weeks. I started by explaining, "I have malignant cells," then graduated to admitting, "I have a hard time saying the c-word, but I need to have surgery," and finally was able to say, "I have breast cancer, and need to go through treatment." Find your own comfort level over time with divulging the "c" word.

How Can I Be Sick? I Feel Great! A Bit of Healthy Denial Is Just Fine.

Your initial response to the doctor's unfortunate news might be exactly this. Sorry, cancer doesn't discriminate, but your response is very typical—denial. You want to deny that cancer could find its way into your busy, fulfilling life, when you are so energetic and strong and feel great. You may have never even had any other "female" health conditions before, so this must be a mistake. Unfortunately, breast cancer doesn't provide any warning until the tumor appears, and even then is not generally associated with any pain or discomfort. So, you refuse to believe that this could be happening to you.

Denial is the first stage of the grieving process of denial, anger, and eventual acceptance. It is a natural human emotional response, and must be balanced between constructive and destructive aspects. Use your denial in constructive ways to keep your attitude positive, to keep your life as "normal" as possible, to refuse to believe that you might die. You are entitled to a bit of healthy denial, and inevitably will move through it to accept it in your own time frame and on your own terms. It is a loss to be grieved—a perceived loss of femininity and sexuality, a loss of a sense of invincibility and immortality, and in the case of mastectomies, a physical loss of part of your body. Nobody can deny you the entitlement to grieve and experience a sense that your own body has betrayed you. However, don't let it become destructive. Don't let denial paralyze you to the extent that you don't seek out advice regarding treatment and hopeful eradication of this disease from your body as soon as possible! And don't hesitate to seek out support groups even if you think you're really "fine" with it.

Come Back Next Month. The Timing Here Is Really Terrible.

Sorry, there's never a good time for cancer to enter your life. You might even jump into high gear, worrying about how you're ever going to fit it into your already hectic schedule. Work is crazy, your kids never get enough of your time, your parents complain they never see you, and you rarely have an adult conversation with your spouse these days. Save yourself the worry. This is the one non-negotiable in your schedule over the next six to twelve months. Accept the fact that cancer will take its place front and center in the midst of your hectic schedule. And hopefully, all those people placing all those demands on you will rise to the occasion and help you manage that schedule.

REACTING TO THE NEWS: IT'S ALL IN YOUR ATTITUDE

You Didn't Cause This . . . and If You've Got to Get One of the C's . . .

Let's make one thing clear. No matter what your lifestyle, nutritional habits, exercise regime, family history, or anything else that you've read about that *might* contribute to cancer, there is nothing you did that caused this. You did not ask for it. It's just one of those mysteries in life that happened. And while you might consider yourself one of the unlucky one-in-eight women that gets breast cancer, it's not as if the other seven escape "home free." There is not one person in this world who will escape having to deal with some type of disease in the course of his or her life. So, the other seven will end up with something else. This cheery idea was pointed out to me by one of my doctors as an attempt at encouragement in one of my tearier moments. Furthermore, as one of my friends rationalized to me, "If you've got to get one of the *C*'s, it's not a bad one to get . . . because it's completely treatable!"

Paternal Genetics: Does He or Doesn't He?

In your quest to come to terms with why you got breast cancer, you'll hear many different opinions on the role of genetics. Is breast cancer hereditary? From whom? While there seems to be consensus and a predominant focus that a history of breast cancer on your maternal side—grandmother, mother, sisters, aunts—places you in a higher risk category, paternal genetics can play an equal role in determining your predisposition to breast cancer. Look for patterns in your father's relatives as well.

Ten Leading Risk Factors

It seems like everything you do, or don't do, eat, or don't eat, or even breathe in can cause cancer these days. Until now, you probably haven't organized your life around how to avoid cancer, and you might have had no risk factors, but you still got it anyway. So, going forward you might want to be aware of the risk factors that you can control so you can manage them to prevent a new breast cancer:

Some Basic Factors You Just Can't Change

1. **Family history.** If it's in your genes, there's not much you can do, except regular monitoring to catch any recurrences or cancers in the other breast in the earliest stages. In the extreme, you might consider prophylactic mastectomy if you carry the genes (see the discussion in Chapter 8, "Five-Year Follow-Up Visits" for overview of genetic testing).
2. **Early menstruation or late menopause.** If you started menstruating before age 12, or went through menopause after 55, the many years of estrogen surges from your monthly

---

cycle may trigger breast cancer, as some types grow and flourish on estrogen.

3. *Childbirth after age 30 or no children.* Hopefully you haven't done your family planning around whether you might get breast cancer, as there are much more important decisions around bringing a child into this world. But late childbearing or not having children is a risk factor because of the continuous exposure to monthly estrogen cycles, without an interruption for pregnancy.

4. *Exposure to radiation.* If you've ever received any form of radiation to the chest area before age 30, say for Hodgkin's disease, you are more susceptible to breast cancer.

5. *Use of estrogen/progesterone.* This increases risk, mostly for lobular cancer.

And Those Over Which You Have Control

6. *Smoking.* If you ever have, just don't, not ever again. You want your life—not breast, lung, or many other types of cancer. Enough said.

7. *Obesity.* Fat cells produce estrogen, a potential nutrient source for breast cancer cells. If you've always wanted that lean, healthy body, now is the time to make it happen, not just for cosmetic, but for very real health reasons.

8. *High-fat diet.* Again, fat consumption boosts estrogen, and the last thing you need after breast cancer is more estrogen. So, stick to a diet low in saturated fats (some monounsaturated fats are fine). You'll also prevent obesity (see the discussion in Chapter 9, "Nutrition: Looking at Food in an Entirely Different Way").

9. *Lack of exercise.* You've been bombarded, ad nauseam, by information on the health benefits of exercise. So you don't need me to tell you any more about how regular aerobic exercise strengthens the immune system to rid your body of bad cells before they turn cancerous (yes, everyone has bad cells; cancer just forms when your immune system can't eliminate them from your body properly). But I will tell you that a review in the *Journal of the NCI* (1/21/98) evaluated a range of studies on the effects of exercise on breast cancer, and reaffirmed its risk-reducing effect in healthy women of all ages.

10. *Alcohol.* There is a growing body of evidence linking alcohol intake to breast cancer, especially heavy use.

Remember, You Are Not a "Cancer Patient."

"You are not a cancer patient. You are most likely a healthy person who has *had* some cancer that was removed and are now fine. Remember that. There is a difference." These were the first words of the first oncologist I went to visit for an opinion. While I didn't ultimately choose him for treatment, I found this extraordinarily helpful mental model to keep me positive and focused. According to him, "cancer patients" are those unfortunate people who must manage cancer until it ends their life at some point. With early-stage breast cancer, the theory is that most women are cured from surgery alone, and they will go on to have long, healthy lives. However, any and all the follow-up treatment recommended is purely "insurance"—or "adjuvant" treatment—so you will hopefully never have to become a "cancer patient."

You Haven't Been Robbed of Your Youth. You've Been Granted Incremental Wisdom.

If, like me, you are young—I was just 35 when diagnosed—one of the emotions you might experience in the initial days of coming to accept your new reality is a feeling that you've been robbed of your youth. Yes, rationally you understand all the doctors' optimism about 90+ percent survival rates for early-stage diagnoses, and you fundamentally believe that you will grow old and live a full life. However, on an emotional level you can't help but think that you have been robbed of your youth, your invincibility. Your body, which you have always taken for granted and considered immortal, has betrayed you. From now on, you must defer to it, honor it, even make promises and negotiate with it. Now you will always remember what it feels like to have had a brush with mortality. Whenever you are contemplating a major life event—your wedding, the birth of your child, watching your children grow up, etc.—never again will you be able to ignore that little voice in the very back of your mind whispering, "Will I be alive to experience it?"

Instead of feeling shortchanged, robbed of your youth, consider that you've been granted a premature wisdom and perspective on life that many women twenty to thirty years your senior haven't grasped yet. You will cherish and appreciate those special life events even more, and remember where they rank in your ever-competing life priorities. It's a gift. Use it wisely. And don't ever lose it.

It's a Very Tough Way to Find Out You Don't Control the World.

It's your diagnosis alone, and try as you might, nobody else's. As many times as you might say, "No, this isn't happening to me," it's not going to walk away from you anytime soon. Just accept it. Then get going at gathering information and making decisions regarding your treatment plan. That, at least, is something you can control. No matter what your occupation, if you work, you get paid every day for making decisions. So, make decisions about your own life with consideration, courage, and conviction. At least you'll feel like you're back in charge.

It's Okay to Have an Occasional Panic Attack.

By the end of the first month into this whole breast cancer ordeal, you will probably be so sick of people reminding you that "Your attitude is everything. . . . Stay positive and you'll stay well." How do they know?!?! Since when did they become experts, especially those people who panic when they break a fingernail? They don't have a magic crystal ball. You feel like telling them to go jump in a lake and leave you to sulk or panic on occasion. That's just fine; it's perfectly okay. If you *didn't* have occasional moments of panic about not reaching your next birthday, not being around to see your children off to college, not enjoying your retirement days, you wouldn't be normal. You might even still be in the denial stage of coming to accept your condition.

Acceptance: It's Amazing How Your Mind Comes to Terms with Reality.

You may experience a slow evolution to acceptance of whatever treatments are necessary to deal with your specific cancer by a unique process of bargaining with yourself. The good news is you always win, and you also come to accept issues when you are emotionally ready to handle them.

I began with an attitude of, "Okay, I want to do surgery as fast as possible, but we caught it early so I won't need anything else, except maybe a little radiation." Then, following surgery, when my doctors started discussing adjuvant chemotherapy because of the size of my tumor and aggressiveness of the cell types, I conceded, "All right, just a little chemo, but nothing too toxic. Make sure I don't lose my hair." And finally, after several opinions from oncologists and the realization and acceptance that this *is* a serious disease that could kill me if I don't treat it properly, my attitude became, "Who cares about my hair, I want my life! Bring in the big guns! Give me the most aggressive chemo you have . . . I'm tough, I can handle it. And by the way, what else do you have in your arsenal that I can do to make sure that this never, ever comes back?!?!"

A Whole New Meaning to One Day at a Time.

If you're reading this book, you are probably a planner, an organizer, just like me. You've often been advised not to worry about the future, just to take one day at a time as it comes. Guess what? It's true. With cancer, that rush to get to tomorrow comes to a screeching halt. Sure you want to get all this surgery and treatment stuff over with and behind you because you might just not feel that great. But beyond that, just savoring today brings a whole new perspective to that old adage. Because you'll never know what tomorrow will bring—either good or bad.

SPREADING THE NEWS: EXPOSING YOURSELF TO THE WORLD

Okay, so you've now broken the news to your cherished "inner circle" as part of the means to help you comprehend the magnitude of this news. So what's next? How do you spread—or not spread, if that's your choice—the news to a broader group of people. To whom do you turn first? Who needs to know directly from you? How do you control the message so the rumor mill doesn't run rampant? Do you even care? How do you manage this entire process without feeling an incredible sense of exposure and vulnerability?

Enlist Your Inner Circle . . . Assign Roles.

In additional to enlisting your inner circle for emotional support (that goes without saying, it's why you chose them), you also want to communicate with them about the very practical, logistical things you might need help with over the next few months. Based on how you think each person might be most helpful, you can assign roles to help you. Some might have the right temperament to accompany you to doctor appointments and consultations, helping to take notes, listening for you when you really aren't hearing, and managing medical records to alleviate you of such administrative headaches. Others might contribute by helping with research and gathering information, which may simultaneously lower *their* anxiety levels, as they become more educated and informed. And others may be best suited to helping to manage your family and life chores, including babysitting, running errands, housekeeping, cooking, etc.

Tread Lightly on Your Partner. . . . He May Be on Overload Right Now.

If your spouse or significant other has momentary lapses of unexplainable or strange behavior, cut him a bit of slack right now. He's acting double, even triple, duty right now, trying to deal with his own emotions and fears of losing you, while also needing to appear strong and supportive of you. Furthermore, if you have children who need caretaking, he also may be taking on a greater share of the burden of handling both their reactions and schedules to lighten the load on you. If at times, he needs to withdraw, get angry, not seem as supportive as possible, let him. Just make sure you keep your communications channels open, to let him acknowledge and validate his feelings. Just as you are entitled to momentary respites from playing the hero, so is he.

Young Kids Are Amazingly Intuitive. Don't Hide . . .

If you have young children at home, they will probably know something is wrong long before you say a word to them. Kids are amazingly intuitive and will just know, so don't hide. Most experts would advise you to be candid and straightforward with information, but not too clinical. Don't explain more than they need to know. Try to be reassuring, but also realistic as they will see straight through sugar-coated stories by the tone of your voice and your behavior and that of other adults around. Since a sense of security is very important to children, try to enlist family members or friends whom they are comfortable with to help ensure their routine stays normal, and your need for medical care disrupts them as little as possible.

However, in the end, you know your children best—their levels of perception, comprehension, and development—and are in the best position to gauge what they can handle. Cancer is such a delicate issue that you might consider enlisting professional expertise through this initial phase. Ask your doctors to refer you to appropriate social workers and/or child psychologists.

. . . But Older Kids May Be More Difficult to Predict.

The older your children are, the less likely you'll be able to hide anything from them. But the more difficult it may be to predict their response to your illness. They may be a terrific source of support and comfort, both logistically and emotionally. Or they may retreat, reeling from having their world turned upside down as you—their source of nurturing and comfort—now need to be nurtured and comforted. Furthermore, the reaction of daughters often becomes more complicated, as they may experience their own fears or anxieties about the possibly hereditary nature of this disease and may feel guilt and/or resentment that they are unsure how to contend with.

Help Your Friends Along. . . . They May Be Waiting for "Clues" from You.

Some of your friends will immediately move into helpful mode and instinctually know what to do to help you. Others, however, may either be paralyzed by the fear of losing you, or simply awkward and embarrassed, and will not know what to do until you offer specific suggestions. And still others will be unable to deal with your diagnosis due to their own insecurities and fears of mortality and will disappear, either temporarily or permanently. You just have to remind yourself that other people's behavior really has less to do with the strength of your friendship than with that individual's own psychological constitution and prior experience with cancer (e.g., they may be terrified because they lost a loved one to cancer). So, for those who do stay in the picture but don't know how to help, tell them. Start with something small, such as picking up a few groceries for you on their way home because you might be too tired. Gauge their responsiveness, and determine whether to ask for bigger favors, such as accompanying you to chemotherapy.

If you haven't heard from people that you'd expect to, call them. Just hearing your voice sounding normal will put them at ease, and also break the ice in the event that they've felt awkward about calling you.

Be Prepared for Stupid Responses from Smart People. (They Really Don't Mean It.)

It's not that people intentionally try to say stupid things. It's just that most people—even those who are highly intelligent and articulate—have no idea how to respond to the statement, "I have breast cancer." Not only does the word "cancer" equate to mortality, but the word "breast" equates with sexuality in our society. What a double whammy. Most people don't know whether to feel awkward, embarrassed, pitying, comforting, or what. Just as you felt an entire range of emotions upon your diagnosis, they will need a minute to collect their thoughts and respond as best they know how. However, you'll find that most people don't collect their thoughts first, so you'll get some awfully stupid responses. Three of my favorites follow (you'll soon have your own list . . . it should make you smile):

- From an acquaintance I hadn't spoken to in a while, who called to ask me to lunch on the day of my first chemotherapy appointment: In response to my statement, "Unfortunately, today I start chemotherapy treatment for breast cancer," he said, "Oh, so I guess you're not available for lunch." No questions about what happened, how I'm doing, or what he might do to help me. He was probably just so overwhelmed, he couldn't respond.
- From a coworker with whom I often lamented that my extensive travel schedule was running me down: "So, do you think the stress of the job and being on airplanes too much caused this?" A naïve, uninformed search for some explanation, some

reason how this could happen to someone as young and healthy as I.

- From someone I had dated, when I serendipitously ran into him (and I knew that he had heard about me through friends but hadn't contacted me): "Oh, hi, Deb, new 'do'?" My reply: "No, _____ [I'll spare you his name], it's a wig, but see, I'm actually getting my hair back underneath!" as I pulled the elastic of my wig away from my scalp and watched the blood drain from his face. I'd never seen him speechless before.

How to respond to stupid comments? Just move beyond them, ignore them. Instead, let the person know that you feel lucky that it's been caught early, that your prognosis is very good, and that you will be fine. Your optimism and attitude will make them more comfortable (plus save them later embarrassment when, in retrospect, they realize how stupid they were). And besides, the critical issue is not how they respond upon the initial shock of the news, but about how they treat you through your entire experience. You might find that people initially eager to help fall by the wayside, while others, who may be shell-shocked at first, are there for the long haul.

Surround Yourself with Only Positive-Energy People.

While there are those that will say stupid things at first, they will accept the shock and move on to be helpful to you in their own ways. However, there are those who never get over the shock, those who can't handle *your* diagnosis. They're worried, upset, and the negative energy of their mere presence brings you down. "Hey, remember, *I'm* the one with cancer!" you want to shake them and scream. Guess what? It's their problem, not yours, and if they can't handle it, get them out of your life. You've got enough to handle right now, other than worrying about other people's emotions. How to do it? One woman I met wrote a letter to her sister, who was driving her crazy because she was living out her own anxieties about the disease and what it might do to their family. She simply wrote that until her sister could control herself and focus on helping the situation, she'd appreciate it if she stayed away. It's a pretty tough way to do it, but consider the experience a filtering mechanism to get the clutter out of your life. Surround yourself with only positive-energy people who will uplift you, people who will be there for you—unconditionally.

Assign a Weekly Medical "Reporter." It Lets You Focus on More Newsworthy Matters.

Once the news spreads of your diagnosis, you will get so many calls that you'll begin to think that AT&T has rerouted their central switchboard to you. It's all very flattering as you realize just how many people in the world care about you and love you, and they are calling to offer support in any way they can. But it can also be very exhausting, both physically and emotionally. Physically, you simply might not have the energy to return all those phone calls, and tell everyone how you are that day. You might just want to rest. Emotionally, you'd rather jump off a bridge than tell one more person how much arm mobility you've regained post-surgery or how low your white blood counts were that week. Eventually, you'll get confused, and won't even remember who you told what. Furthermore, it will continue from the moment of diagnosis through to the day you remove your wig once your hair has grown back (if you lose it). So what to do? Some people find it helpful, especially early on, to assign a weekly medical "reporter," someone you appoint on a rotating basis. This person is the point person to whom you can refer anyone who wants to know about your medical status. That way, you are freed from "reporting" your status repeatedly, and can turn your discussions to more interesting matters of what else is going on in your and your callers' lives.

Have Several Versions of Your Story: The Hollywood Fluff, the Reader's Digest *Condensed Version, and the Great American Novel.*

Not everybody needs to know your exact situation. But you probably need some people you can tell every nitty-gritty detail to help you cope with it. So you might determine who needs to know what as follows:

- *Hollywood fluff.* For those on the periphery of your life, those you see only sporadically, your party line might be something like, "Oh, I had some surgery and I've been recovering, but I'll be fine." You're not lying, but simply glossing over some of the unpleasant details, and focusing on the hopefully happy ending, just like many Hollywood movies. I used this one when I attended a school reunion just three weeks after surgery, and the week before I started chemotherapy. When people I hadn't seen in five years tried to hug me, I politely replied, "Please don't hug me. I recently had surgery around my arm, and am still in some pain." Their response was quite often, "Really? You look terrific for just having had surgery!" It made me smile.

- **Reader's Digest *condensed version*.** This is the right take for casual friends and relatives with whom you are friendly but not too close. These are people you see on a regular basis, who need to know what you've been through in order not to expect too much from you during this time. You just won't be your normal energetic, dependable self. However, there might be reason to be more guarded with this group, so stick to the facts, and focus on making these people comfortable that you are handling this well and will soon be back to normal. Your employer and coworkers probably fall into this category.

- *Great American novel.* Reserve the nitty-gritty details of what's happening to your body for your inner circle, for those few people who are living this day in, day out with you. These are the individuals who you know are strong enough to handle it and be there for you for the long haul. They're also the ones who will tell you candidly if they need to step away from the situation temporarily. Often, family members, especially spouses, are so emotionally involved in your cancer that they need space from time to time. Let them breathe. They'll be back when you need them.

Take the Lead at Work: Shatter in the Workplace the Three Myths of Cancer.

Take a leading, proactive role at work from Day One. You will not only become a role model for your ability to manage your way through any crisis, be it work or cancer, but you will provide a valuable education for those with preconceived myths about cancer patients at work. The three most frequent myths—two of which extend far beyond the workplace—are:

- *Cancer is a death sentence.* Since people have so many misconceptions about survival statistics, they may inadvertently take a patronizing attitude toward you, trying to shield you from excess work, office politics, or whatever else. They may even pity you. While intentions may be good, they are often founded on false fears. Besides, it should be up to you to determine how much work you can handle right now, what issues you want to address, and what protection you might need. In fact, since work may be one of the few sources of stability in your life right now, it might be very unsettling to feel like you are being left out of the loop on what may be important issues and decisions.
- *Cancer is contagious.* People may avoid you based on their own irrational fears of contracting the disease. Interact with such people on relevant work issues as appropriate, and reinforce the positive aspects of how you can work together. You might be so helpful to them that they'll just forget their fears and understand that cancer is *not* contagious.
- *Cancer is a drain on productivity and efficiency.* The pervasive myth is that cancer patients are a drain on short-term productivity (e.g., taking a lot of sick days) and that over the longer term they are not good "investments" to train, promote, and develop. The reality is that cancer patients and survivors are often more productive and work harder, because they have clarity on what's important in their lives, and how work fits into those priorities. They focus on the essential elements of getting their jobs done, particularly when trying to balance the job demands with treatment schedules.

Discrimination based on such false perceptions can be very subtle, but very real, so by maintaining your composure, a positive attitude, and a focus on the business issues at hand, you will demonstrate your strength, reinforce your capabilities, and provide information and awareness that will alleviate coworkers' concerns. Furthermore, you will hopefully help to make the workplace a bit more comfortable for the one out of two men, and one out of three women who will be diagnosed with some type of cancer in this century.

The Only Work Pressure on You Is You. With Planning, Everyone Else Will Understand.

Although you may want to help shatter the myths of cancer in the workplace, if you need a break, give yourself a break. Let them worry about the business, while you worry about yourself for the near future. Don't put any undue pressure on yourself to perform right now. After all, as much as you want to be strong and a role model at work, you do have a life-threatening disease (even though you try not to remind yourself of this fact). Your employer survived just fine before you arrived, so they'll do just fine without you for a short time, if that's what you want (unless you're self-employed, and then, hopefully, you've hired good people).

There are many ways to give yourself a break if you need it. With a bit of planning to make your employer comfortable that your work will be covered, you might arrange for:

- *A leave of absence.* If you work for a company with more than fifty employees, your employer is legally obligated to grant you up to twelve weeks of unpaid leave under the Family Medical Leave Act (FMLA) of 1993. (See discussion in Chapter 7, "Balancing Work.") While this information may not be actively promoted by your HR department, they are required by law to alert you of it should you inform them of your need for medical treatment. Determine if you have other sources of income so that you might be able to afford time away.
- *Revised schedule or reduced working hours.* Some type of part-time arrangement; fewer hours per day or less than five days per week. While part-time status is not mandated by FMLA or ADA, you might negotiate this with your employer.
- *Short-term disability benefits.* Depending on your employer's benefit structure, you may be eligible for short-term disability, which provides you with a percentage of your salary for a defined period of leave, usually between six and twelve weeks.

- *Less travel.* Reducing any work-required travel will lessen fatigue and enable you to keep treatment appointments (remember, these are nonnegotiable).
- *Delegate projects.* Lean on your coworkers and staff a bit more than you might normally—you'll be surprised at how willing they will be to step in and rise to the occasion.

Of course, your ability to continue to keep a "normal" work schedule throughout will depend on your physical energy level. And if you take time off, you might even get a "welcome back" party. Now you know how much you were missed!

Strength Does Not Equal "No Tears."

So, up to now, you've been the heroic role model of an exemplary patient at work. What happens when you just can't maintain that façade any longer, on those days you feel like your world is crumbling around you? What to do? Permit yourself to cry at work; just do it in a quiet moment behind closed doors. As much as we hate to admit it, the typical workplace is very male-oriented, which means "No Tears," but you wouldn't be human—or at least female—if you couldn't show a bit of vulnerability on occasion. You might even ask for extra help now and you deserve it. After all, if you've been a good performer, the company should consider itself lucky to have an employee so dedicated as you that you're worried about disrupting the workplace with your emotions.

Activate Your Civil Rights

The decision about how, when, and if to tell your employer about your cancer diagnosis is often shrouded in a dense cloud of emotions, which include fear, anxiety, and relief, as well as some very practical concerns about job security and your right to privacy. Furthermore, whom do you tell? Your boss, the human resources officers, or only a trusted coworker who might help manage some of your workload should you need relief? Relax a bit. If you choose to be candid and straightforward about your diagnosis, you will "activate" an umbrella of civil rights—a group of federal and state laws that offer protection for your position and provide you with "reasonable" accommodations if you are able to perform the essential functions of your position, should you need to adjust your work schedule to get through your cancer experience.

The two most relevant programs include the **Americans with Disabilities Act (ADA)** and the **Family Medical Leave Act (FMLA)**. (See Chapter 7, "Balancing Work," for details on each program.) Just imagine that you have bundles of these rights burning holes in your pockets, screaming to be pulled out and utilized to protect you. The few simple requirements? Your employer must be **aware and knowledgeable** of your condition, and you must be able to perform the essential functions of your position. Begin an ongoing, **nonconfrontational** dialogue by officially communicating to your HR department as soon as you realize you might want or need time off from work (basic surgery will require at least some time off). Provide just the **basic** facts about your situation. Don't volunteer too much information or detail, as you never know how information can be misconstrued and where it may end up. For example, if you are seeing a social worker or psychiatrist to deal with the emotional impact on you and your family, your employer only needs to know that you may need to miss work for regular medical appointments associated with your cancer. **Document any conversations and commitments your employer has made to you—in writing.** If you don't, you may regret it when you need to draw on your rights and you failed to activate them.

Hint: Practice first. Rehearse what you're going to say with family or friends because you might be nervous. Also, be specific about what you want from your employer. They have rights too, and will need to balance the potential financial burden of your partial or full absence from work, with accommodating you as best they can under the legal framework.

A Final Thought: Making Others Comfortable Is Fine, but Remember to Take Care of Yourself First.

Look back at the past few days or weeks, and give yourself a pat on the back for what you've accomplished so far. You've exposed yourself to the entire world—or at least you feel that way—and you've maintained your composure and strength, while quelling the anxieties of others. Whether you've been proactive at work dispelling myths about cancer in the workplace, or comforting friends or family who might fear your mortality or their own, bravo! Now remember that *you're* the one with cancer! There's a fine balance between making others comfortable so they are there to support you, and weeding out those whom you might not want around right now. Your mental and physical energy should be focused on you now, not them.

CHAPTER 2
Swinging into Action

You may not believe me until you're deep in the thick of it, but getting together a game plan for how you're going to deal with your cancer experience goes a long way toward regaining a sense of control over your body and your emotions. Once you've picked yourself up off the floor after being whacked with that tidal wave of a diagnosis, you realize there is something very empowering and reassuring about taking action to manage your situation. This chapter addresses:

- The process and sources for *Gathering Information,* whether you become your own chief researcher, or you delegate to a family member, friend, or someone in your inner circle.
- *Establishing Support and Coping Mechanisms* to help you through your breast cancer experience.
- Recommendations on *Building Your Health Care Team,* including an overview of all the medical professionals and specialists involved, and how to get them most effectively working for you.

GATHERING INFORMATION: BECOMING AN INSTANT EXPERT

You Can Research Forever, but Faith in Your Doctor Is the End Goal.

Depending upon the specific circumstances around your diagnosis, how it unfolded, and when you received critical pieces of information, you may need to do research at several different times during the progression through your cancer experience. For example, I went through two phases. First, after receiving the results of my biopsy that showed malignant cells, and an initial consultation with my breast surgeon, who recommended a lumpectomy, I sought out a second opinion. I also did my own research on the pros and cons of lumpectomy versus mastectomy to feel comfortable with the lumpectomy recommendation of both doctors I had seen. (See Chapter 3, "Evaluating Your Options" for more on how that decision gets made by the medical community.) Then, once I received the pathology report that detailed the results of my lumpectomy surgery, with its implications for follow-up treatment, I sought out opinions from oncologists as to various chemotherapy options.

Each of you will have a slightly different experience as to when you need to gather information, for example, if you are having a mastectomy and have to consider immediate versus delayed reconstructive surgery. However, for simplicity's sake, I will discuss the entire research and information-gathering process here in this section. It might turn out to be a few pages that you come back to time and time again.

The critical point to remember is that while you are the ultimate decision maker as to what does or does not happen to your body, in the end, you must have faith in and be comfortable with your doctors. You can do research until the cows come home, but your doctors have dedicated their lives to this topic, so you will never match their expertise, experience, and insight. All you can hope to do is gain a basic understanding to feel comfortable with their recommendations. If you aren't comfortable, ask for explanations until you are. If you don't receive satisfactory explanations in jargon-free, nontechnical English, maybe you should consider another doctor, one with whom you can develop a stronger rapport.

Time Doesn't Stand Still, but It Will Pause for a Few Weeks.

This research phase may seem more ominous than attempting to read an entire semester's syllabus two days before the final exam. You're paralyzed as to where to even begin, and you're sure that the cancer will grow exponentially inside you by the hour unless you have surgery tomorrow. Relax a bit. Most of the medical research suggests no variation in survival rates or treatment efficacy as long as you begin treatment within four to six weeks. So, take a couple of weeks to get all the information you need to feel comfortable with a decision, and then let it settle in for a week or so, as you'll be living with this decision the rest of your life. By all means, don't dally, but consider it nature's reprieve, or time well spent, so you're intellectually and emotionally ready when treatment begins.

Rationalize the Mortality Statistics: Consider It Healthy Denial.

No matter what stage your diagnosis, Stage I or Stage II, you will become terrified when you start to look at the mortality statistics associated with each. Overall, the statistical probability is that you will make it to the five-year survival mark, but you sure don't want to be one of those statistics that doesn't. Furthermore, you are not a statistic but a person. Statistics are necessary landmarks that doctors use to make treatment decisions among thousands of patients, and they may not be reflective of how your particular case unfolds.

Find your own coping mechanisms to convince yourself that you will fall into the survivor group. What I did was take comfort in my otherwise healthy lifestyle. I convinced myself that the minority of women in Stage I or Stage II who don't make it to the five-year survival mark must be smokers, drinkers, overweight, already 98 years old, or had some other chronic condition that contributed to their poor prognosis. I also reminded myself that any study I read must be at least five years old to have had sufficient data to publish, and the medical world knows more every year about treating breast cancer—and a lot more than they did five years ago. In fact, according to annual statistics compiled by the National Cancer Institute and the Centers for Disease Control, 1996 was the first year in more than thirty years that the death rate from breast cancer actually declined, attributed to more wide-spread screening to identify cancer early on, and more effective systemic treatment at the early stages. So, the statistics five years from now—when they're important to us—will look even better. Consider whatever rationalization you come up with your own form of healthy denial.

Read, Educate Yourself, and Ask So Many Questions That You Drive Your Doctor Nuts.

The single most influential determinant of getting the best care and treatment is *you*. Educate yourself. Read everything you can handle, at whatever stage you can handle it. (See pages 39–44 for some helpful reference books and association materials.) You'll know when you are emotionally ready to read the harsher, more clinical material. Some may be too scary too early on. Put yourself on a somewhat level playing field. Write a list of questions to ask your doctors. You're paying a lot of money for their expertise, so educate yourself enough to hold an intelligent discussion. Tap all the knowledge you can and utilize it well. Then, together the two of you can decide what's best for your otherwise healthy body, your disease state, and your emotional state.

Find a Collaborator If You Need Some Heavy Lifting.

If you find that you just can't focus on or absorb any reading material right now, or you just don't want to do it, enlist the help of someone from your inner circle to sort through research for you and bring you only the information relevant to your decisions. Some women find this an excellent way to involve their spouses in the process. If the man in your life fits the stereotype of being more comfortable solving problems than dealing with emotions, research is perfect for him. It will make him feel that he is helping to solve the problem in a rational, practical way. Alternatively, some women turn to family members or friends who are medical professionals, and most likely have access to resources and can grasp medically technical language. Or if you know someone who is a survivor, she may be able to jump in and even provide research shortcuts as she already knows where to look.

There's Much More to a "Second Opinion" Than Just an Opinion.

If you don't get the information you seek or satisfactory responses in consulting with an oncologist as to how to treat your disease, get a second opinion (and sometimes even a third, as a tiebreaker if there is a discrepancy between your first two). A thorough, comprehensive second opinion will most likely include the following:

- A review of your complete medical history, even beyond breast cancer (to determine if there are any considerations that might affect treatment decisions).
- A full physical exam.
- A review of the "slides" of your tumor, or microscope slides containing slices of the cancerous tissue removed, which are evaluated by a pathologist.
- A review of any X rays or imaging studies, such as mammograms or sonograms, by a breast radiologist.
- A detailed proposal for a treatment plan.

. . . But a Thorough Opinion Results from Providing a Thorough Medical Portfolio.

To aid your doctor in giving you the most comprehensive, detailed opinion possible, you must be well prepared. Make sure you bring all relevant medical reports, including:

- All pathology reports and slides (pre- and postsurgery).
- All radiographic materials, such as mammograms, X rays, CAT scans, etc.
- All lab reports from routine tests, including blood tests.
- Any reports from other medical conditions that you think might affect your treatment (if in doubt, bring it).

If possible, get as much information as you can to the doctor ahead of time in order for him or her to review before your appointment. Offer to fax copies of written reports a couple of days ahead. But *never* send original films or slides. Keep those in your sight at all times. Pick them up from the originating institution and carry them with you to any other consultation.

Be Aggressive. . . . Isn't That What Sports Coaches Always Tell You?

If you've ever competed in any sports in your life, your coach has always told you to "get out there, be aggressive, just do it." (Yes, Nike has made many millions off those last three words.)

And now you have your health care team most likely telling you to "Be Aggressive." Why? Why would they want you to undergo un-necessary trauma if there's a chance you were cured with surgery? Fast-forward five years. Don't you want to be able to look back at your treatment protocol and say to yourself, "We did everything possible at that time to make sure that my cancer would never ever come back"? You'll live every successive day of your life in comfort. And even if you should face a recurrence, you'll have the comfort of knowing that you did whatever you could to prevent it. You'll never have to live with the guilt of "I should have . . ." or "I wish the doc-tors had told me to do . . ." So, since everyone involved wants you to have a long, full life, the treatment recommended to you may seem aggressive, but will optimize your survival chances.

Beware of Information Overload. Know When to Stop Reading.

At different points in your journey through this experience, you will hit your "information overload" threshold. Your mind will start spinning, you'll experience confusion rather than clarity on deci-sions, and you'll start terrifying yourself by thinking that every neg-ative aspect of this disease definitely applies to you. You might even start to blank out and not be able to absorb any more. It's your brain's protective way of signaling to you that enough is enough.

Overload Relief: Find a Mental Parachute for Quick Bailouts.

You know you've just reached your limit. You just can't think about, talk about, or deal with your cancer for one more minute. Find an emotional escape mechanism, a mental parachute that lets you bail out at a moment's notice. One caveat: What might have worked for you in the past might not be appropriate for this time in your life. Under normal circumstances, I am an avid athlete and outdoors person, which I very much utilize as my escape from everyday life. However, in the midst of my surgery and treatment period, I found that I couldn't be as adventurous as I normally might (plus I couldn't be too far from a hospital). So, my escape became reading—everything from inspirational outdoor adventures, such as expeditions up Mt. Everest, to books about art and architecture. Everything except breast cancer. Find what works for you, what makes you feel good and inspires you, be it reading a juicy novel, yoga or meditation, music, jigsaw puzzles, knitting . . . anything you can pick up at a moment's notice. When you have to come back to reality, you'll find yourself mentally refreshed and recharged.

Warning: You May Not Die of Breast Cancer, but the Reference Books Might Crush You.

I admit to stealing this line from the infamous television character Murphy Brown (remember her?), who exclaimed it while standing in her office buried by reams of computer printouts and books on cancer when she was initially diagnosed with breast cancer. It's true. At some point, sooner or later, you will have done all the research you need to determine what's best for you. You'll know when you reach that point, as you'll be both mentally and physically exhausted. And regardless of the lists of pros and cons you've made for various alternatives, you'll know in your gut what you want to do, even though it may seem terrifying. Don't let that instinct be crushed by all those reference materials.

Take a Deep Breath and Plunge In. The Sooner You Get Going, the Sooner It'll Be Over.

When you've exhausted your tolerance for information gathering and come to that conclusion about what's best for you, you have to just get going with treatment. Just like stepping off a high dive into a swimming pool, you never know exactly how you're going to land and how cold the water will be, but eventually you'll surface. The important thing is to just get going. Remember, you should start treatment within four to six weeks of surgery. This is enough time to gather the information you need to feel like you're in control of your decision, to recover a bit from surgery, and to "strike while the iron is hot" (so said one of my doctors) to get the most impact from treatment. Take the time you need to feel comfortable, but don't delay. Just plunge in, and before you know it, it will be over.

A Special Note on Alternative or Complementary Medicine: Save It for Later?

You may be wondering about if and/or how to incorporate alternative or complementary medicine into your treatment regimen. This is a very personal decision—to be made in conjunction with your doctor—based on your belief systems, religious persuasion, faith in the traditional medical community, and a host of other factors. I used a blend of both at different times. I relied solely on traditional Western medicine to get me through the immediate crisis—making sure that cancer was gone from my body, through surgery, chemotherapy, and radiation. I made this decision partly based on my own beliefs and partly at the recommendation of my health-care team, who were concerned about the potential for herbal remedies to interfere with the effectiveness of my treatment. However, I have decided to pursue some alternative therapies in my postcancer program—including nutritional changes, herbal programs, consistency of exercise, etc.—for both physical and emotional reasons. Not only do I try to keep my body as healthy as possible, but by taking active steps to enhance my overall health, I feel that I have at least some semblance of control over my body and my life again. Should I ever get a recurrence, I won't look back and blame myself for not doing everything in my power to prevent it. (See Chapter 9, "Alternative Medicine," for a discussion of basic alternatives.)

Instant Expertise:
Useful References and Organizations

Since any other cancer book that you open will most likely contain extensive appendices listing information sources and suggested reading, I'll be brief here. Here are just a few of the most accessible, informative sources I've found:

Books/Publications

• *Dr. Susan Love's Breast Book,* by Susan M. Love, M.D.

This everything-you-wanted-to-know-about-breasts-and-cancer-but-were-afraid-of-and-afraid-to-ask 600-page tome is the "bible" of clinical breast cancer books. Although she is somewhat controversial politically, and it comes through in her writing, Dr. Love's easy-to-understand language, and non–jargon-laden descriptions of complex medical issues is a must-read before you meet with surgeons and oncologists to discuss treatment alternatives. At times it may terrify you, but you'll be glad you got through it to know what questions to ask your doctors, and to be able to understand their responses to make informed decisions. It also contains appendices with extensive listings of additional resources, references, suggested reading, and listings of both national cancer centers and regional support organizations. Then, return to this book for some hope and a smile.

• *MAMM: Women, Cancer and Community*

349 West 12th Street
New York, NY 10014
Phone: 888-901-MAMM (for subscription information)
Web site: www.mamm.com

Directly from their Web site: "MAMM is the women's magazine dedicated to providing the necessary tools to live healthier and happier lives with a cancer diagnosis. MAMM is for anyone whose life has been impacted by breast or reproductive cancers, including partners, family members and coworkers. Each issue provides the latest treatment updates (including emerging findings about alternative and complementary therapies), inspiring profiles of women who are survivors, and insightful coverage of controversies, politics and culture as viewed through the unique prism of cancer diagnosis." An annual subscription to this bimonthly magazine is less than $15, and well worth the helpful advice and inspiration it provides. Consider it as ongoing chapters of a book like this one, with new advice and helpful hints every other month!

Organizations

- ### National Alliance of Breast Cancer Organizations (NABCO)

  9 East 37th Street, 10th floor
  New York, NY 10016
  Phone: 212-889-0606, 800-719-9154
  Web site: www.nabco.org

  A network of over 375 organizations, NABCO is the leading nonprofit central resource for breast cancer. It's a wealth of information and resources to guide you through your decision-making and treatment phases, but has also been my best source of staying informed since. While the mass media may tend to hype studies as "the next cure," NABCO's publications offer practical discussion and analysis of breakthroughs and new developments in the treatment of the disease. They offer the answer to, "What do the results of this study *really* mean?" and "What are the experts' attitudes toward practical, rather than purely scientific, applications?" Your health is worth the nominal annual subscription fee, which entitles you to an extensive resource list, newsletter, and special conference news highlights of breast cancer medical forums and conferences.

- ### National Cancer Institute (NCI)

  Bethesda, MD 20892
  Phone: 800-4-CANCER (Cancer Information Service)
  Web site(s): www.cancernet.gov or www.nlm.nih.gov (for the U.S. National Library of Medicine's MEDLINE and other online services)

  As one of eight government agencies that comprise the National Institutes of Health, NCI is funded through the U.S. Department of Health & Human Services. Their nationwide Cancer Information Service (CIS) is a free public service education network that has trained staff to answer your questions, send you relevant written materials, or refer you to resources in your local area, including medical facilities, home care assistance programs, and support groups and services (both emotional and financial). Information is also available via their CancerFax® computerized service, by calling 301-402-5874 and following instructions. Or you can access their Web site, which can also be your gateway to Internet breast cancer information, as they provide a directory of "Useful Links."

Regardless of how you contact NCI, you'll have access to their database, Physician Data Query (PDQ), the most detailed, timely data relevant to your specific cancer available anywhere. Just provide the details of your specific cancer—cell types, stage, tumor size, etc.—and they'll send the latest on treatment protocols, side effects, prognosis, relevant clinical trials, and research programs. There are two versions—one for doctors, one for consumers. Neither is uplifting reading, but discussing them with your doctor will reassure you that you are on the leading edge of treatment.

- **American Cancer Society (ACS)**

  National Office
  1599 Clifton Road, NE
  Atlanta, GA 30329-4251
  Phone: 1-800-ACS-2345, 1-800-395-LOOK (for Look Good, Feel Better® Program only)
  Web site: www.cancer.org

With chapters in most major cities, the volunteer-based ACS is one of the most widely known cancer organizations. Since ACS deals with all types and stages of cancer, its services are extensive, but some of the written publications can be a bit generic (better to stick with books specific to breast cancer or publications provided by your doctors). However, ACS efforts specifically for breast cancer include:

- *Reach to Recovery.* This is a one-to-one visitation program for women who have just been through surgery. An ACS-trained survivor offers assistance with the physical and emotional issues that the newly diagnosed woman must address. It's like having a new friend who really does understand exactly where you're coming from.

- *Look Good, Feel Better.* Cosponsored by the National Cosmetology Association and the Cosmetic, Toiletry and

Fragrance Association, the premise of this program is that women can benefit from the psychological "lift" of looking their best. This one-time, two-hour session teaches you how to "mask" the ugly side effects of chemo and radiation (e.g., hair loss, skin changes). Not only will you be given a wig if you need one, and good tips for wig care, but you'll go home with a big box of cosmetics from leading companies like Estée Lauder, Chanel, Lancôme, and others!

■ *TLC Catalog.* This seasonal catalog offers essential products for women coping with effects of the disease, including hats, scarves, hairpieces, and bathing suits and prostheses for women with mastectomies. Call 1-800-850-9445 to order.

● **The Breast Cancer Fund**

282 Second Avenue, 2nd floor
San Francisco, CA 94105
Phone: 415-543-2979 or 800-487-0492
Web site: www.breastcancerfund.org

The Breast Cancer Fund (BCF) was founded in 1992 to raise awareness and fund cutting-edge projects in research, education, patient support, and advocacy. Its mission is to eliminate deaths from breast cancer in our lifetime, and make sure that women living with breast cancer receive the best available care and support. Emphasizing quality of life for women living with breast cancer, they focus on such issues as early detection programs, the value of exercise during treatment, psycho-social programs for patients and families, integration of complementary techniques with traditional medical treatments, and research in areas such as investigating less toxic treatments or the potential impact of the environment on the development of breast cancer.

One of their more visible programs to raise hope, awareness, and funding is "Climb Against the Odds," in which a group of breast cancer survivors climb some of the world's highest mountain peaks (which have included Mt. McKinley and Mt. Aconcagua to date). The motivational message is that you can make it through breast cancer just as you can make it to the top of a mountain—one step at a time.

- *SHARE*

    1501 Broadway, 17th floor
    New York, NY 10036
    Phone: 212-719-0364 or 212-382-2111 (for hotline)
    Web site: www.sharecancersupport.org

    This New York–based volunteer organization is a unique, non-profit self-help support organization for women with breast or ovarian cancer and their families and friends. SHARE's services include information hotlines, peer-led support groups, public education, advocacy, and wellness programs. Visible on a national basis, SHARE's work enables women to make informed decisions about their medical care and treatment, and contributes to a broader awareness regarding research, prevention, and early detection. With its extensive and broad membership, SHARE's programs run the gamut, including special programs for young women, parenting after breast cancer, alternative medicine and nutrition, meditation and visualization, and information on leading-edge medical breakthroughs. Even if you don't live in New York, it's a very helpful network to tap into.

- *National Coalition for Cancer Survivorship*

    1010 Wayne Avenue, 5th floor
    Silver Spring, MD 20910
    Phone: 888-YES-NCCS or 888-650-9127 (toll-free direct line)
    Web site: www.canceradvocacy.org

    Founded by and for cancer survivors, NCCS is a national grassroots network. Its mission is to lead and strengthen the cancer survivorship movement, to empower cancer survivors, and to advocate for policy issues that affect survivors' quality of life. NCCS serves as a clearinghouse for information on services and materials on survivorship. A sampling of the useful publications available from NCCS (some for a nominal fee, others free) include: "Working It Out: Your Employment Rights as a Cancer Survivor," or "What Cancer Survivors Need to Know About Health Insurance." Their Web site also contains a useful section called "CanSearch: Online Guide to Cancer Research." In addition to general oncology-related Web sites, it suggests several breast cancer–specific sites.

- **Y-ME Breast Cancer Support Program, Inc.**

  212 West Van Buren, 4th floor
  Chicago, IL 60607
  Phone: 800-221-2141
  Web site: www.y-me.org

  Y-Me provides information and education programs for patients, as well as a telephone hotline staffed by trained survivors who can share concerns and exchange information. Y-Me also maintains a wig and prosthesis bank.

- **CancerCare**

  1180 Avenue of the Americas, 2nd floor
  New York, NY 10036
  Phone: 212-221-3300 or 800-813-HOPE (4673)
  Web site: www.cancercare.org

  CancerCare's offices are located primarily in the Northeast United States, but they offer a wide range of services to cancer patients and their families nationwide via a toll-free hotline, teleconferences, and their Web site. Among the free services CancerCare offers are: individual counseling and support groups, information and education, and access to financial resources and assistance. While CancerCare offers guidance for all cancers, they have special programs unique to different types of cancer. For example, their Web site contains numerous prerecorded teleconferences on breast cancer topics ranging from "Sexuality and Breast Cancer" to "All You Wanted to Know about Tamoxifen."

Web Sites Can Be Helpful . . . But Three Caveats About the Internet

Yes, the Internet can be a fabulous source of information, but it can also be dangerous. Its helpfulness is the wealth of the most up-to-date information, free of charge, that can be searched for on very specific topics (e.g., surgery, hormone treatment) directly from the medical community. Aside from the Web sites associated with the organizations mentioned above, I won't even attempt to offer recommendations on helpful Web sites, as new sites emerge daily. However, don't feel compelled to go "surfing" immediately. And remember that chatting with total strangers is not the same as reviewing medical articles on Medscape.

Consider one woman who stayed awake all through the night she was diagnosed, gathering material on treatment options to discuss with her doctor. By morning she had terrified herself, convinced that any treatment would leave her with permanent, debilitating side effects that she refused to endure. She exclaimed to me, "Did you know that there's something called 'chemo-brain' where you lose your memory?" I calmly replied, "That sounds suspicious. Did it ever occur to you that the woman you were 'chatting' with on-line may have been eighty-eight years old and a victim of Alzheimer's?" "No," she replied. "Maybe I am being silly." With that said, I give you three caveats about chatting on-line:

- *Caveat 1: You never know who's on the other end.* When you go on-line to talk to people about cancer, or any subject, you have no idea who is at the other end, and what their physical, mental or emotional state may be. People enter the world of cancer with very different health histories which may have nothing to do with the cancer challenge at hand.

- *Caveat 2: Every person and case is different.* When you start discussing cancer therapies with other women, there is an immediate tendency to compare yourselves, to go running to your doctors sure that they are missing something because all other women have been told to do something that you haven't. Resist the temptation. Every single case of cancer is different and you have no idea why one doctor recommended what he or she did. This is true when you've actually met, but even more so on the Internet, when you've never even seen the woman!

- *Caveat 3: The focus may be more on problems than answers.* Most people who take the time and effort to sign on are generally seeking solutions to their own problems rather than altruistically offering advice about how to sail through challenging times. Approach Web sites and chatrooms a bit irreverently, and keep your focus on finding answers, not unearthing new worries.

Nope, You Didn't Choose It, Sister, but You've Just Been Initiated into a Special Sorority.

It's never too late to gather helpful information, even when you're well into the treatment phase. Regardless of any ambivalence you might have about not wanting to be around other people who are "sick"—no, not me, you think—get to know other women going through this. They're the only other people in the world who really understand exactly what you are going through. Plus, they're a great source of information. When you go for your first chemotherapy treatment, you might be afraid to talk with other women there. Don't be. They are all seasoned "pros" and they are just waiting to give you helpful pieces of advice, comfort, and encouragement. Go ahead. Talk to them. It will make *them* feel better to know they're helping you, and you might walk away with some helpful hints.

ESTABLISHING SUPPORT AND COPING MECHANISMS

Brace Yourself for the Emotional Roller Coaster . . .

In the ups and downs of an individual's emotional life, any significant changes—sometimes even good ones—may cause an increase in stress, worry, or anxiety which can throw you onto an emotional roller coaster. Particularly during breast cancer, it is very common for women to seek out help—from a variety of sources—at any or all phases: (a) at the shock of diagnosis, (b) during the seemingly endless routine of treatment, and (c) upon the completion of treatment, facing the uncertainty of returning to "normal" life.

To be perfectly candid, I found the most emotionally difficult time to be after it was all over. I had put my head down and plodded my way through, simply focusing on my day-by-day physical changes and needs. But then it was over. Doctors were no longer monitoring me weekly. I had done everything medically possible to prevent the cancer from recurring. And my phone no longer rang several times a day with friends and family calling to find out how I felt and what they could do for me. All that was left to do was go back to my life and wait . . . and hopefully live a full life until I'm an old woman of 90.

. . . And Beware of Triggering Events.

While the whole experience of breast cancer is probably a significant enough change for all of us to ride the emotional roller coaster, there are moments of particular vulnerability, or "triggering events" that can set off feelings of panic, worry, and undue anxiety. They can happen at obvious times, such as birthday or anniversary celebrations (anything that marks the passing of time and realization that we're all mortal) or upon entering a treatment facility or hospital to go for chemotherapy (which brings back memories of past visits). Or they can happen at very unexpected moments, perhaps even something as seemingly innocuous as scheduling an appointment. So, brace yourself for them, call on your coping mechanisms, and ride them out, knowing they are normal and should subside.

Don't Be Bashful about Asking for Professional Help.

If you find yourself in any type of elevated emotional state for more than a few weeks at a time, or reeling from emotions that prevent you from functioning, then it's time to seek individual counseling. Prolonged feelings of being overwhelmed, helpless, out of control, angry, depressed, or paralyzed about making a decision deserve the attention of a trained professional. Find someone who specializes in the issues associated with cancer, and better yet, breast cancer. Many women—especially those who are independent, self-sufficient, and used to a great sense of control and mastery over their lives—find that this small task of asking for extra help is excruciatingly difficult. Why? By nature, women are not programmed to ask for help, but are raised to be the nurturers, the caretakers. So when we need help ourselves, we enter unfamiliar territory, uncertain about where to turn and what to do. If you feel a sense of hopelessness, loss, and inability to make a decision, do not hesitate to call any of your doctors and ask for help.

Find a Role Model like Gracie the Taxi Driver.

In the midst of my chemotherapy treatments, I was graciously invited to spend a restful, relaxing weekend on Block Island—a tranquil, rustic summer resort area off the coast of Newport, Rhode Island. My hosts greeted me at the ferry terminal, and we jumped in a taxicab back to their home. During the ride, I happened to mention the book I was considering writing. Out of the blue, from the front seat, our (female) driver exclaimed, "Honey, I don't mean to interrupt, but I had breast cancer when I was 37, and I'd buy your book today!" When I inquired as to her age, Gracie proudly informed me she was 83 years old and still driving her cab. Find a survivor role model like Gracie, someone you can look to for inspiration and hope.

Ever Heard the Expression, "God Only Dishes Out Adversity to Those Who He Knows Can Handle It"? Enough Already. Pick on Someone Else."

While I'm not a terribly religious person, there definitely seems to be somebody upstairs doing a great job of targeting me. Little does he know that my "reserve" barrel of strength is running very low. In fact, for ten years prior to my own diagnosis, I was preoccupied with trying to find some treatment, some hope, for my mother's chronic, life-debilitating illness, multiple sclerosis. So, when breast cancer arrived on the scene, in a very twisted, sordid way, I almost felt as if I had been prepared to handle it. Yes, the multitude of options for treating breast cancer today can be overwhelming. But consider yourself fortunate that there is so much attention and so many resources being funneled toward eradicating our disease versus more limited options for other conditions.

Do you feel like you're another lucky target? Step back and consider any adversity you've faced in your life to date. Determine what qualities in you it might have drawn out, how it might have given you the fortitude to get yourself through breast cancer. And be sure to tell that somebody upstairs that you've had enough dished out to you for a while!

Analyze Your Coping History to Discover Effective Patterns.

Although you may never have faced anything as traumatic as breast cancer before, all of us have had to cope with some type of life-changing event or crisis over the years. It might have been a move to a new city, a job change, or even a transfer to a new school as a child (yes, sometimes childhood behavioral patterns can offer great clues as to your intrinsic personality strengths, before you were influenced by societal expectations). Ask yourself a few of the following questions: Am I an information gatherer, or do I misconstrue information so it scares me? Am I better talking about things, being very open to everyone, or keeping my circumstances and emotions held close to the vest, to share only with my inner circle? At what stages in my decisions do I feel comfortable talking about them, early on to gather information, or not until I've come to a conclusion? What kinds of actions have worked in the past to make you feel better, and what has tended to make you feel worse? If you are still confused and unsure, ask someone who knows you well to help you. Another perspective may bring surprising insights.

Three Ways to Cry (or Not to Cry)

There are times to cry and times when you just can't let yourself cry. So here are a few pointers on managing your very volatile emotional state:

- *Let it all out.* Just walk down the street, or drive down the road with tears streaming down your face. It doesn't matter if people stare at you. They're strangers and you'll never see them again. Or alternatively, someone might ask you what's wrong, and you'll make a new friend.
- *Hold it in until you get _____.* You fill in the blank: home, back to your office behind closed doors, into your car, with your partner or friend, whatever. Just promise yourself a time when you know it will be safe to cry. It will keep you composed if you know you can break down later.
- *Suck it up.* When you just can't now and don't know when, take a deep breath, think about your favorite vacation destination, force a smile, and change the subject.

Your Family? The Rock of Gibralter Has Soft Spots Too.

Although family members are often a terrific source of support, remember that they, too, are human, and will experience (or deny) your disease in their own very personal way. So, there may be times when their emotional states and your needs aren't in sync, when they can't give you what you need at the moment. Don't push it. Although the institution of family should be the strongest foundation you can rely on, this rock of Gibralter also has soft spots in its constitution. So turn elsewhere for the moment—to friends, support groups, etc.—and reconnect with those individuals later. Ask *them* how they are doing and coping. Remember, cancer is a family experience.

The Delicate Dance of Intimacy Continues. What Do We, I, and You Need?

Once your partner is through his own initial shock of your diagnosis, you may need to have a frank discussion about reorganizing your roles and perhaps the entire family structure for the time being. One of the most common pitfalls in relationships is that people stop talking, and this is especially true when breast cancer is involved. Women may feel guilty about "burdening" their significant others with their physical and emotional changes, and their need to be taken care of right now. And their partners don't want to scare them with their own feelings, or exhibit too much discomfort with the physical changes. Keep the intimacy with open and honest dialogue. However, you should develop some ground rules about what to talk about, what *not* to talk about, and when. Don't, for example, discuss your fears of mortality just before bedtime (unless you want a sleepless night). Some people prefer to avoid heavy decision-making conversations at dinner, keeping mealtime enjoyable and uplifting.

Regardless of what other issues are on the table, you need to develop clear answers to the question, "What do we need to do together to cope with this, what do *I* need specifically and what's best for *you?*" Address this at several levels, from emotional to physical to day-to-day logistics of living. Be candid about your need for distance or closeness, for the independence and self-sufficiency required to triumph over this disease, tempered by your vulnerability and need for nurturing right now. Don't expect just to shift the burden to your partner, for example, in household chores or caring for children. He might need some help himself, and together you'll need to develop a solution, be it recruiting additional help from family and friends, or hiring professionals to handle housekeeping, grocery shopping, or other chores that might just overwhelm you right now. And expect the answers to shift as you progress through the experience. Keep the communication channels open to renegotiate when appropriate.

That's What (Girl) Friends Are For.

Have you ever heard that expression and not really known why it was such a classic? Now you will. If there was one theme that I heard over and over from single women, married women, all women regardless of their involvements with men, it was that "my friends were there." No matter how helpful or supportive their spouse, significant other, or any other man, at the core of this experience, it was really their girlfriends who were the most consistent, solid, stable supporters. Many women complimented the men in their lives for being wonderful and supportive. Yet they also stated in no uncertain terms that it was only another woman who could put herself in their place, empathizing with the entire range of emotional issues—body image, sexuality, motherhood/parenting—that breast cancer wreaks havoc with. One woman even started a bulletin board of all the cards and notes sent by her girlfriends during her hospital stay, and then continued it through treatment. It served as a daily visual reminder of all those women who were there for her.

Remember, you may not be able to predict who will or won't be there for you. Many women mentioned the reappearance of old friends—some breast cancer survivors themselves—despite being out of touch for prolonged time periods. And all mentioned those who fled, as we discussed earlier. True friends step forward, and others fade. Learn from this experience.

What Is a Friend? A Very Special Job Description

I've always considered myself lucky to have so many interesting, varied, dynamic, considerate, caring, and just plain fun friends in my life. But it wasn't until I was diagnosed that these friendships were ever actually tested—rocked to their very core, pared down to the essence of going that extra mile in putting someone else's needs ahead of your own. I learned a lot about human nature, about the fundamental character of many individuals, and about which friends would come through with flying colors, and which would fall by the wayside to the periphery of my existence. It's wasn't always easy, and it wouldn't be my choice of a way to do it, but many of my friendships have deepened and been enriched because of it. What I learned is that a friend:

- Is willing to hold your hand while a nurse injects your chemotherapy into your veins.
- Volunteers to drive you to the emergency room on a holiday weekend.
- Tracks your weekly white blood counts closer than you do.
- Thinks your wigs look better than your real hair (or tells you if they don't).
- Sends you get-well cards on a regular basis, long after the others have stopped flowing in . . . just to make you smile.
- Tells you inspiring stories of other women who have been there and are fine.
- Protects you, until you are ready for it, from sad news about women who didn't make it.
- Remembers that you still are a person with many facets even though you now have breast cancer (there are more interesting topics to discuss than your most recent doctor visit).
- Is there through all the bad times as well as the good.

The Hidden Advantages of Being a Single Woman.

I want to say a few words of hope about life as a single woman. You may feel overwhelmed by managing this disease on your own, and wonder why you have been dealt this hand to manage alone. Think again, as there are actually several aspects of being alone that can be quite advantageous. Among other things, singleness offers:

- *An unspoken beacon for help.* Since your singleness signals the entire world that you're alone, different people will surely step in to help at moments you need it. Contrast this to a woman in a half-baked relationship or, worse yet, a relationship that was troubled even before the cancer diagnosis. The world assumes that since she is married or involved, she is not only being taken care of physically (e.g., someone to accompany her to doctors' appointments), but has a solid foundation of emotional support as well. This is rarely the case. And even when she is being taken care of physically, it is only a terrific relationship that sails through the traumas of a cancer journey. Many women in relationships admit to being very lonely through this experience.

- *A more even distribution of your "burden."* Upon my diagnosis, I was shattered that I had not yet found that life partner to be by my side through this journey, and be my sounding board for decisions that could have had lifelong consequences. However, about three months into my treatment, I realized that it wasn't so bad. As I progressively felt weaker and not as much myself, I realized that in a way I was lucky not to have the guilt of burdening any one individual with my day-to-day experience, and make him endure it with me. Instead, I was able to "distribute" the burden among several people, in more tolerable increments, so nobody became too overwhelmed or unable to escape at times.

- *A character screen for future relationships.* You may not feel like dating during this time in your life as you're preoccupied with other things (you never know, though, as one woman I encountered met her husband in the radiation waiting room, the son of another breast cancer patient). However, once you are ready to return to the dating world, consider cancer a very effective screening mechanism that tests the character of any man you may potentially bring into your life. Unlike married women, whose spouses get the real-time battle conditions, you have the luxury of revealing your cancer history as the relationship unfolds, whenever you feel the time and situation are appropriate. Both the immediate and the longer-term reaction of your date will give you glaring insight into the strength and depth of his character. If he runs away, you probably didn't want him anyway. What would happen when life's next big crisis emerged? While it sounds like a daunting challenge, most women also mentioned that their own attitude when they broached the subject greatly eased a potentially awkward situation. Many even used humor. One woman was invited to her date's house for dinner, and when he was telling her about his dog, and how she somehow had lost one nipple from a surgical procedure, she introduced the subject by responding, "Oh, so your dog and I have something in common!"

Finding a Support Group Is like a Shopping Expedition.

The cardinal rule of support groups is they are not all alike. Group dynamics and effectiveness will vary dramatically, based on a variety of factors, especially the composition of its members and the underlying philosophies of the sponsoring organization. For example, some groups are exclusively breast cancer, others all types of cancer, others consist of the same age or stage of disease. Furthermore, the main focus and the types of participants attracted may be affected by whether the sponsoring organization is a hospital, a breast cancer advocacy organization, or even an alternative health program.

So, think of your search for a support group that works for you as a shopping expedition. Sometimes you'll hit on that perfect outfit on the first try, and other times you'll need to scour the entire mall before you find something to fit you. And always try before you buy. If you decide that you'd like to participate in a support group, but don't click initially, don't give up on the first try. Give it two to three sessions before you determine that it's time to move on to try another group. Try to look for a match in terms of your primary diagnosis and age group. And finally, be wary of any group of highly politicized women. You should be in a support group right now to be able to discuss your stress and anxiety openly, to get assistance with coping mechanisms, and to find comfort. You do not need to be saving the world from breast cancer (at least not yet).

Create Something . . . Anything.

Even if you never thought of yourself as creative, you are. You're involved in creation every day, but you just don't take the time to recognize it and cherish its life-affirming effects. In your daily life, you are busy creating—raising children, cooking meals, tending a garden, building an organization, solving work problems, or engaging in a host of other activities. Stop and appreciate your efforts.

However, upon a cancer diagnosis, many women take their creativity to a whole new level, by tapping into pieces of themselves they'd never known before. (I never thought I'd be an author!) Maybe it's driven by a very subtle or real fear of dying, and we just want to make sure we've lived a fulfilling life. Regardless of the outlet, create something. It doesn't matter whether it's an artistic endeavor such as taking up photography or dance or painting, or simply sculpting each new day in your children's lives. Value it as a tremendous emotional outlet in your journey toward healing.

Just Escape, Nature's Way.

I have heard many different women, in many different ways, describe some type of relationship with nature and the out-of-doors as being important to their healing. The more active women, particularly some who had been lifelong runners, continued their running (albeit at a more moderate pace) as therapy, visualizing every step as squashing cancer cells, and every breath as breathing in clean, healing air and new life. Other, less active women mentioned that just being outside, alone with nature in beautiful surroundings, was spiritually consoling, comforting, and peaceful. Even if you can't physically get to some place you want to be, visualize it until you *can* get there. On some of my longer, darker days, when I was stuck in the summer heat of New York City, needing to be close to the hospital, I just imagined what I would do first on my next trip to visit my family in Vermont. Would I take a walk or a bike ride? Would I play with the dogs in the yard? Would I simply sit on the back porch, surrounded by greenery, look up at the mountains rising ahead of me, and listen to the wind chimes, the hummingbirds, and other voices of nature? It didn't really matter. It was my outlet, and I knew I'd be there soon.

Schedule a Minivacation into Every Day.

Over and over again, you'll hear, "Be good to yourself." If there ever was a time in your life to be a bit selfish, it is now. In fact, be sure to "schedule" one small part of each day for something that gives you pleasure. It might have something to do with your new-found creativity. Or it might just make you feel good—taking a relaxing bath, preparing a great meal, reading a wonderful book. Not only will it be a diversion from the regimented schedule you need to tolerate, but it may also provide a sense of mastery, or maintenance of control over your own life (when doctors and others will be calling the shots more than you may be used to).

Emulate Scarlett O'Hara. Use Procrastination Productively.

There's a wonderful scene at the end of the movie, *Gone With the Wind.* Rhett Butler is gone, Scarlett O'Hara's child is dead, and our heroine simply proclaims, "I'll think about that tomorrow." Don't completely deny the issue, just delay it. What a beautiful coping mechanism. Pick a specific time to worry, later. It's like putting your worries in a box to open another time. And when it gets to that time, you have two choices. First, you can keep your promise to yourself and spend a few minutes processing your worries and fears, determining how to handle them. Or perhaps by the time your worry appointment approaches, you've forgotten what it was that you were so distressed about!

BUILDING YOUR HEALTH CARE TEAM: A CRITICAL ELEMENT IN WINNING THIS GAME

In the midst of dealing with probably the most imminent life crisis you have faced to date, the last thing you need to do is feel like a Ping-Pong ball, being bounced back and forth between doctors, who tell you, "Well, you'll have to talk to _____ about that issue." Wrong! What you want is a team of health care experts who all work together regardless of their institutional affiliations or specialties. It is not your role to be translator, arbitrator, or diplomat. They should be talking to each other as needed, and you should simply be one more member of that team—actually the lead member, because it is you who decides who needs to talk to whom when, and ultimately decides what will be done to your body and when. This section provides some guidance on how to go about building and coordinating that all-important health care team.

Finding a Doctor Is Easy. Choosing One Is Harder.

By the time you read this, you have regretfully already arrived at the diagnosis of "cancer." And the person who accompanied you to this destination was probably either your general physician or your gynecologist (perhaps through their mammography technicians). If you've felt good about your doctor-patient relationship over the years, by all means, use him or her as the foundation for building your team. They should have a network of peers and other specialists at their institution (and throughout the community) with whom they regularly work and to whom they will refer you. However, just because your doctor refers you to someone doesn't mean that you must accept treatment from that person. You have the right to find your own alternative, or simply to talk to other experts to verify the reputations and recommendations of those you've been referred to.

So, how do you find other breast cancer specialists? Don't underestimate your network of friends and family. Ask everyone you know, even if you think they've never known anyone with breast cancer. Talk to other survivors and call breast cancer organizations to get referrals. The world gets very small quickly, and certain names in your community will start coming back to you repeatedly. Those are the doctors you want to consult.

If you exhaust the friends and family circle, inquire at your church or synagogue, as these institutions often have survivor support groups you might be referred to, and part of your clergyman's job may involve affiliations with local medical institutions.

The Basic Players: Surgeon, Medical Oncologist, Radiation Oncologist . . . but No Indian Chiefs?

You will very quickly be overwhelmed by how many people suddenly become interested in your body. Below is a list of specialists who might be involved in your case, depending on your particular circumstances and chosen treatment. At different phases, different doctors may play the role of "lead" doctor on your team, as I've indicated here. At the very least, identify one of your doctors—perhaps the one you are closest to emotionally—to help you manage this team through the entire ordeal as a sort of cocaptain.

- *Surgeon (breast or general).* Depending on the size of the community in which you live and the availability of breast surgery specialists, you might choose a breast specialist or a general surgeon who has simply done a lot of breast surgery. He or she will be your "lead" doctor through what is frequently the initial phase of cancer, the surgery. However, in some cases, if he or she determines—from the biopsy or mammogram, perhaps—that the tumor is rather large, then your surgeon might ask you to consult with an oncologist to determine if chemotherapy is warranted to shrink the tumor prior to surgically removing it.

- *Plastic Surgeon.* If you undergo reconstructive surgery either simultaneously with or subsequent to a mastectomy, you should choose a plastic surgeon who will work hand-in-hand with your breast surgeon. Not only will they be sharing the operating room if your reconstruction process is begun during the mastectomy surgery, but they will need to agree on which type of reconstructive surgery is most appropriate for your body type and desired outcomes (more later on your choices). If you choose simultaneous reconstruction, you need surgeons who work from the same hospital. However, if you decide to reconstruct subsequently, either months or years later, your plastic surgeon choices are basically unlimited.

- *Pathologist.* Although it's not up to you which pathologist your surgeon chooses to work with, the pathologist is still a critical member of your team. He or she will be the one to perform several tests on pieces of tumor removed to determine the aggressiveness of the cancer type and the extent that it has or hasn't spread through your body. This pathology report will be the basis for what your oncologists recommend as the course of subsequent treatment, if any. (See Chapter 5, "A Note from the Oncologist: Breaking the Code: Reading a Pathology Report.")

- *Medical Oncologist.* A medical oncologist is an expert in the use of a variety of "modalities" used to treat cancer, including chemical and hormonal therapies. This is the doctor who will determine and oversee your chemotherapy regimen, if it's required. While your surgeon will have oncologists to whom he or she can refer you, you are completely free to choose your own oncologist. When the surgery phase is complete, your surgeon will essentially hand you over to your oncologist, who will become your "lead" doctor.

- *Oncology Nurses.* The nurses who actually administer your chemotherapy treatments will be some of the most valuable sources of information you can find in terms of the practical "stuff" to get you through this. Why? Because not only are they very special people, who must be very compassionate and comforting to do what they do, but they also sit for hours with patients to whom they are administering drugs, and patients often talk to pass the time. They'll express their fears and hopes, and sometimes they'll share very useful advice that can be passed along to you. If there is a nurse that you particularly liked and found helpful, do not hesitate to request her for subsequent treatments.

- *Radiation Oncologist.* A radiation oncologist is the doctor who plans a program of radiation therapy (i.e., local treatment of breast cancer with high-dose X rays), using physics to determine how to effectively radiate the entire breast for maximum impact on any remaining cancer cells, while minimizing damage to the healthy tissue. Although your medical oncologist can refer you to a radiation oncologist, there will be others to choose from, especially if you are at a large medical center. Ask around. The nurses, receptionists, other patients in the waiting room all may be able to give you information about the reputations and personal styles of the radiation oncologists.

- *Radiation Therapist.* Radiation therapists are the technologists who run the machines that administer your daily radiation treatment. There might be a few different people operating the machine you are assigned to, and although you do not choose them, they will quickly become your friends, because you will be seeing them every day for six or seven weeks.

- *Psychologist or Psychiatrist.* Depending on your emotional state at various stages of your recovery, you might want to take advantage of the mental health resources the hospital can provide. Do not be afraid or ashamed to ask your surgeon or oncologist for recommendations if you feel yourself paralyzed by fear, falling apart, or generally unable to cope. Remember, your doctors should be looking at you as an entire individual to be treated . . . that's why there's this big team! Therapists affiliated with the hospital should be particularly adept at handling cancer and survivorship issues. If you need help, get it, no matter when.

- *Social Worker.* Believe it or not, there are a wide variety of social and economic aspects to breast cancer that you may have never imagined until it was thrust upon you. Since you may be overwhelmed right now simply adjusting to your diagnosis and physical changes, you might rely on a social worker to identify extra sources of support for you. A few of the things they can help you with are finding support groups, securing community assistance for home health care, and even help in managing the insurance and financial aspects.

- *Nutritionist.* The more we learn, the more we know that good nutrition is a key weapon in the war against breast cancer (so important, in fact, that there's an entire section later on how to eat well for the rest of your life). Ask your doctors if there's a nutritionist on staff who can review your diet, (1) while you are undergoing treatment, as there are certain foods that might help you tolerate chemotherapy and its side effects better than others, and (2) following treatment, when you will want an ongoing nutrition program that will strengthen your immune system.

- *Geneticist.* If you come from a family with a history of breast cancer, you might want to consider genetic testing before you make any treatment decisions. If you are a carrier of BRCA1 or BRCA2, the breast cancer genes, and are at high risk for recurrence, development of cancer in the other breast, or ovarian cancer, you might consider more aggressive surgeries, such as mastectomy, or even bilateral mastectomies, removal of both breasts, as a preventative measure. If you have daughters, you might start monitoring them more carefully at an earlier age, and have them join a preventative education program (e.g., maintaining a lifestyle that will minimize risks). However, think very carefully about genetic testing, as there are a host of ethical, legal, and insurance implications should such information become part of your publicly available medical history. Ask yourself if there is anything you would do differently from what you're doing today if you discovered you carried the gene. If not, don't bother to see the geneticist.

- *Gynecologist.* Your gynecologist should be informed and have copies of all your medical reports. If your hormones have been affected temporarily by chemotherapy (e.g., menopausal symptoms such as hot flashes or irregular or absent menstrual periods), your gynecologist is the one who might be able to help restore your reproductive cycle to normalcy. Also, once you've had breast cancer, he or she might want to monitor you more carefully for other types of reproductive cancers (see Chapter 8, "Longer-Term Issues: The Aftermath").

Use Your Gynecologist for Perspective . . . Your Reproductive Historian.

The role of your gynecologist on your health care team deserves a special mention here. While he or she is really not directly involved in managing the breast cancer treatment experience, you may find that your gynecologist turns out to be the doctor you rely on the most. Many women find they use their gynecologist as a counselor, the one they can come back to at important crossroads to put all the information from specialists into context, and to be a sounding board to help make decisions. After all, your gynecologist was there before you were introduced to all these specialists under the stress of the cancer crisis at hand, and will be there for you once the experts disperse. He or she knows you as a person, knows your history, helped you with your family planning or any other issues associated with the female life cycle. Your gynecologist can be your thread of continuity before, during, and after your cancer experience.

Interview Your Doctors. Make Them Earn the Privilege of Treating You.

It is your decision about which doctors to use, but everybody will want to put in their two cents: "He cured Aunt Sylvia of her rare blood disease." (Yes, but I have breast cancer.) "She is the best in the world." (Yes, but she practices 3,000 miles away and I can't commute that far.) Listen to everyone's input; take seriously only that of your inner circle (that's why you've chosen them, because you trust them). Then, make your own list of what's important to you. Among other criteria, my own personal list included doctors who were:

- Compassionate and empathetic.
- Honest, straightforward, and informative; not patronizing and/or holding back information.
- Considerate of me and my needs as a whole human being, not just a cancer tumor.
- Viewing me as a unique individual with a treatment plan for me and my needs, not just deliberating over which of their current clinical trials I might qualify for.
- Fact-based and clinically rigid, but also willing to use their gut instinct to determine how best to treat me as an individual.
- Leading edge, both as an individual recognized as an expert in his or her specialty, and as part of a leading institution.
- Well versed in breast cancer issues.
- Accessible, who could be paged or called twenty-four hours a day.

While these were some of my criteria for my entire medical team in general, there were other criteria more specific to each individual specialist.

When It Comes to Oncologists, Choose the Person First, Then the Institution.

Choosing an oncologist to treat you is perhaps one of the most important decisions. It is the doctor with whom you'll spend the most time over the next year, and will see regularly for five years. Your surgeon will finish his work and be gone except for periodic checkups. Your oncologist will be your five-year friend. Don't necessarily choose one of the NCI-designated "comprehensive cancer centers" across the United States just because you feel that you should, or you live near one. Choose an oncologist who meets your criteria list *and* with whom you feel comfortable, someone you will want to visit ten years from now just to say hello and celebrate your ten-year survival anniversary. You should, however, be comfortable that he or she is associated with a high quality hospital.

Make Sure Your Doctors Communicate. Otherwise, You'll Feel like a Ping-Pong Ball.

Once you've assembled this unwieldy team of experts, you need to make sure they continue to communicate throughout your treatment process. Otherwise, instead of concentrating on yourself and feeling as good as you can, you'll feel like a Ping-Pong ball being bounced from one to another and will stress yourself needlessly. A few things you can do to help facilitate communication among the team include the following:

- Keep meticulous notes each time you meet with a doctor, including topics discussed, questions asked, and recommendations made.
- Have copies of all major reports with you at all times in case the doctor with whom you are visiting just misplaced something (e.g., biopsy results, pathology report, recent mammogram).
- Have your nurses help by reporting anything unusual to the doctors they are working with.
- Have your doctor send copies to the rest of the team of any written reports submitted to your file.

Ask for a Free "Trial Visit."

One way to reduce your anxiety about the entire treatment process is to be comfortable in your surroundings. Ask to see exactly where you'll be treated, for radiation, chemotherapy, or both. Is the staff friendly and reassuring? It the environment light, uplifting, and comforting or harsh and clinical? If you can imagine yourself coming there on a regular basis, you'll be less intimidated and more comfortable with your entire health care team.

Create Your Team Log Book, and Become a Meticulous Recordkeeper.

As soon as you can, get a two-inch ring binder with divider sections, and set it up as a log book for all interactions with your health care team. It will also be of tremendous help when you need to deal with financial and insurance issues. Among the sections might be:

- *Team roster*—address, phone and fax of your doctors, and their assistants.
- *Notes*—from consultations and conversations with your doctors. You can refer back to them if you are confused about anything they told you, and perhaps save yourself a call to their office.
- *Test results*—copies of any important test results or reports such as mammograms, pathology reports, etc.
- *Questions*—an ongoing list of questions to ask your doctors during your next visit (unless they are urgent . . . then call immediately).
- *Symptom tracking*—if you are tracking any symptoms associated with treatment such as nausea to report back to your doctors.
- *Financial statements*—keep copies of all medical bills from doctors and hospitals, whether they were sent to you or submitted directly to your insurance company. Also keep copies of all Explanation of Benefit (EOB) statements from your insurance company.

Rules of the Road for Family, Friends, and Other Participants

Just a short introductory note: At the end of each major section of this book, we want to offer some quick, easy "rules of the road" for anyone accompanying a newly diagnosed woman through her breast cancer journey. Too often, you feel helpless, awkward, and unsure where to start or what you can do for her. But hopefully, these "rules of the road" will pave the way a bit more smoothly for you too. This first section offers you some perspective on how to react to those three dreaded words: "I've got cancer." What do you say? How do you treat her? How might you digest this news yourself? And what can you do that might be most helpful right now?

- **Listen. Be a mirror for her emotions.** This is the best thing you can do for a woman who has just been told she has breast cancer. Start now, and listen to her along her entire journey. She will go through the full grieving cycle from denial to acceptance, and you need to be along for the ride. By listening, and playing back to her what you just heard her say, you will help her clarify her own thoughts and feelings. And sometimes, just the act of verbalizing a thought will help both of you realize that it's a ridiculous, unfounded fear that you are using to terrorize yourselves!

- **Don't tell her how to feel.** Listen and reflect, but don't ever tell her how to feel. Don't presume, don't dismiss her thoughts and fears, and don't push any emotion under the rug as too trivial or unwarranted. A reaction of "Oh, don't worry about that, everything will be fine" not only makes you seem patronizing, but who gave you the crystal ball? What she feels, she feels, and she will feel worse if you don't acknowledge it.

- **Help create her own reality.** During these initial stages of shock and grief, she may not necessarily hear, or be able to comprehend, everything her doctors are telling her. She also may not be able to do a lot of research or read about breast cancer without assuming that the worst suggested outcome is her destiny. Help her out. Provide another set of ears to listen to the health care team, and offer to read anything she might not be able to stomach right now. Then create some context for her. Give enough of the facts to paint the reality of the situation; don't gloss over tough issues or feel you need to protect her in any way for her specific situation. But do spare her the anguish of the dismal outcomes that may be completely irrelevant to her case.

- **Allow yourself shock, grief, and momentary distance.** Just as you don't want or expect her to be a twenty-four-hour-a-day hero, you shouldn't be either. Give yourself time and permission to acknowledge your own feelings and fears either to a confidante other than her, or simply to yourself. When you need some time away, literally or figuratively, reassure her that it doesn't mean you love or care about her any less.

- **Ask, don't guess.** Ask her to tell you exactly what she needs when. It's never easy to read people, and especially not in the midst of a cancer crisis. Cancer is a time for clarity and forthrightness.

- **Remember what keeps you a family (if appropriate).** Your normal roles or burden of responsibilities may shift until she gets through treatment. In fact, you may feel overwhelmed and confused about this institution called family that's encountered a sudden upheaval. Stay focused on those values that are at the core of what keeps you a family, including love, caring, consideration, honesty, and above all, commitment and perseverance. When it's your turn for help, she'll be there.

- **Be a strategic messenger.** You can be a tremendous help when it comes to spreading the news to others. Consider yourself her unofficial press agent. Ask her if there's anyone you can call for her or if there's anyone she doesn't want to deal with whom you can protect her from. Also, if there are other family members or friends who may need to be shielded from this news—perhaps because they are going through a crisis of their own and couldn't handle it right now—help her protect them as well.

- **Be an informed, not a sensational, medical advisor.** Generally, only the patient has the vested interest to learn nitty-gritty details of her own disease. However, it helps greatly if you can do some basic homework as well. Learn enough about breast cancer to be able to talk with her intelligently. You'll spare her repeating the explanation she gave to the twenty-nine other people who have asked the same question before you. Plus you might even bring her new information—but please be judicious. Not everything is relevant or authoritative, so leave at home the details of which treatment seemed to have cured Aunt Matilda of stomach cancer, or the latest hype about how shark cartilage can cure cancer completely.

- **Offer inspirational role models.** If you know of other women in her life situation (e.g., married with young children, young and single, recently divorced, older and alone) who have been through breast cancer and are fine, offer them as role models. Offer to put her in touch with them to provide advice and support. Just by knowing that others like her have "been there" will make her feel better. There really is safety in numbers.

- **Get to know her health care team.** Among those of you in her inner circle of family and friends, one person should be responsible for getting to know her entire health care team. It may be her spouse; it may not. Pick up the phone if she needs help getting her questions answered. Look for and point out any inconsistencies in treatment recommendations or communications gaps across the team.

- **Remind yourself that appearances are often illusionary.** As part of your shock and initial denial of her diagnosis, you may find it hard to believe that she's actually sick. After all, she may *look* healthy and strong, in fact, better than ever! Remember that the ravages of a cancer diagnosis and treatment don't always show, so she may look a lot better than she's feeling inside. Temper your optimism and encouragement with a periodic reality check of how she's *really* feeling. Keep the communications channels open.

PART II

SURGERY

CHAPTER 3
Deciding on Surgery

So, you've come to terms with your diagnosis, pulled yourself together, and have begun to put together a strong health care team that you believe in. The first decision you will most likely encounter is what type of surgery you will have. (In a small minority of cases, women require chemotherapy prior to surgery to shrink the tumor.) This chapter offers perspective on the various factors that go into the surgery decision, including:

- *Evaluating Your Options* with your surgeon to determine the best medical, physical, cosmetic, and emotional results for you, and
- *The Financial and Insurance Implications* of various surgical alternatives, and what you need to do to maintain financial security and continuing insurance coverage through the surgical phase and beyond.

EVALUATING YOUR OPTIONS: THE BEST RESULTS FOR YOU

Lumpectomy or Mastectomy: Is There Anything Else on the Menu?

Nope. These are the two types of surgery. Which one your doctors recommend, or whether they offer you a choice, depends on many factors, including:

- *Type of breast cancer.* For the two most prevalent types—infiltrating ductal or infiltrating lobular carcinoma—a lumpectomy may suffice, since these types are usually contained within one portion of the breast in a clearly delineated tumor. However, for other types that tend to be spread throughout the breast tissue, a mastectomy may be mandatory.
- *Absolute size of tumor.* The larger the tumor, the more likely a mastectomy will be required, and will most likely offer a better cosmetic result.
- *Location of tumor(s).* If the tumor is located in a place that would diminish a lumpectomy's cosmetic results (e.g., around or beneath the nipple), a mastectomy might be the preferred alternative. Additionally, if there are multiple tumors spread across the breast tissue, a lumpectomy may not be feasible.
- *Size of tumor relative to breast size.* If you are small-breasted with a fairly large tumor, a mastectomy will more likely provide the better cosmetic results. If you are large-breasted, removal of the tumor by lumpectomy might not even be noticeable, or might be significant enough that you'd be left uneven compared with your other breast, in which case a mastectomy with reconstruction might be a better option.
- *Other health issues.* You may not be a candidate for lumpectomy if you are unable to have radiation for a variety of other, unrelated health reasons. For example, if you have certain collagen vascular diseases or skin disorders, you may or may not be a candidate for either radiation or reconstructive surgery due to potential complications.

Taking into account all these factors, your surgeon will propose the best course of treatment for you. Sometimes he or she might offer you a choice, and sometimes the recommendation might be strongly directed to one or the other alternative. Some women will opt for a mastectomy even though their doctors say that lumpectomy will suffice, because it provides them with maximum emotional comfort. Regardless, you must make the final decision, and it has to be one or the other.

Ask to See Samples, and Variations.

While this is more appropriate for mastectomy patients, any woman should feel free to ask her surgeon to see samples of his or her work. No kidding. Surgeons are used to this. You have every right to know what your chest will look like, either when you awaken, or several months down the line with completed reconstruction. Your surgeon should be willing to draw diagrams, show photographs, and perhaps even provide you with references of other women who would be willing to talk with you about their surgical experience. Be sure you understand exactly what type of surgery your surgeon is recommending. Mastectomies can range from "simple" to "modified radical" to a "quadrantectomy," based on the amount of tissue and muscle removed across the breast and chest wall area. Another means to learn more is through a support group, as many women find that other members are willing to share experiences, and perhaps even showcase their scars. Don't be bashful.

Several women recommended a book called *Winged Victory* by Art Myers, M.D., which artfully captures all types of breast surgery in ways that clinical photos do not. Call 619-221-0340 to order directly, or order at your local bookstore or via Amazon.com.

A NOTE FROM THE SURGEONS

R̽
Mastectomies and Lumpectomies . . .
A Historical Perspective

The first published report of the radical mastectomy appeared in the medical literature as far back as 1894 in a paper by William Halsted, an American surgeon. These early mastectomies were extensive procedures, involving wide "excision," or removal, down to the ribs, usually with a skin graft from the thigh, and always with complete removal of the axillary (or underarm) lymph nodes.

The next eighty-some years saw a gradual diminution in the extensiveness of the surgical approach. By the early 1980s, the less extensive modified radical mastectomy was the preferred approach, due to less disfiguration and fewer complications. However, in 1981 the lumpectomy began to increase in prevalence, with the National Cancer Institute (NCI) publication of clinical trials that demonstrated that lumpectomies had survival rates equivalent to the more extensive mastectomy procedures. In a lumpectomy, the tumor is excised, with a "halo" of surrounding normal tissue, along with axillary lymph nodes. By 1995, a *New England Journal of Medicine* published the results of a ten-year study comparing the survival rates of women with early-stage cancer who underwent either a mastectomy or a lumpectomy followed by radiation. The survival rates were equivalent. These data have held up in recent trials.

In order to be a candidate for a lumpectomy, one needs to have a relatively small tumor in a location that permits an excellent cosmetic result. Lumpectomy is preferred by most patients and surgeons as well, but the size of the tumor in relation to breast size, and the location of the tumor (involving or close to the nipple), might make mastectomy the best choice.

It is important to remember that a lumpectomy is almost always followed by radiation treatment. An interesting recent approach is oncoplastic reduction surgery for large-breasted women, which combines a wide lumpectomy and reduction in the size of both breasts.

Which surgical approach to choose can be a difficult decision, and must take into account many factors. Clearly, discussion with your surgeon will guide you toward the best decision for you. Two similar women with similar tumors may undergo different operations for a variety of medical, clinical, cosmetic, psychological, and practical reasons.

So What Are These Lymph Nodes, and Why Do They Have to Be Removed?

Regardless of what type of surgery you undergo at some point during the operation your surgeon will remove a sampling of lymph nodes from your underarm. Lymph nodes are part of your lymphatic system, which is responsible for removing toxins and cleansing the body.

Technically referred to as an "axillary node dissection," the removal of ten to twenty-five lymph nodes provides significant information to the oncologist to determine what type of additional treatment may be required beyond surgery. The theory is that if breast cancer is going to spread to other parts of the body, it will do so by traveling through either the lymph nodes or the bloodstream. And since the lymph nodes from the chest area all channel through the underarm area, before dispersing out to the body again, the surgeon can remove a sampling from that channel to determine if any cancer has spread beyond the chest. If there are no cancer cells identified in the lymph nodes, then the doctors may assume that the cancer was contained locally, meaning it has not spread beyond the breast. Alternatively, if there are cancer cells in the nodes, then doctors may treat the cancer more aggressively, as they want to kill those cells that have traveled beyond the chest so they don't settle into other organs and start growing.

A NOTE FROM THE SURGEONS

℞

The Sentinel Node Biopsy

In the not-too-distant past, a diagnosis of breast cancer meant removing most, if not all, of the axillary (armpit) lymph nodes. In individuals with no suspicious findings on physical exam, sentinel lymph node biopsy (SLNB) is now the standard of care. By identifying and removing the first lymph node that the tumor would spread to, oncologists and surgeons can accurately stage the disease without removing excess tissue. This significantly reduces the operative time, the need for drains, the risk of lymphedema (arm swelling), and the likelihood of hand or arm infection.

A slightly radioactive isotope and/or a blue dye is injected into the breast. These substances travel via the same pathways (lymphatic channels) as tumor cells and get stuck in the first (sentinel) lymph node in the pathway. The blue "hot" node is removed first and tested for cancer cells (frozen section or quick assay) by the pathologist while the surgeon is performing the lumpectomy or mastectomy. Testing this node will be greater than 95 percent accurate in representing the remaining lymph nodes. Only if the sentinel node is found to contain spread of disease are additional nodes removed.

Wading through the Three-Phase Mastectomy Decision Process.

If you are faced with a mastectomy, you will quickly learn that no two mastectomies are alike, just as no two women's bodies are identical. Based on a combination of emotional and physical or anatomical factors, a patient must wade through an additional set of decisions to determine the optimal solution for her mind and body. This complex decision might be broken down into three more "digestible" phases:

Phase 1. To Reconstruct or Not to Reconstruct: Now or Later?

You will first need to decide whether you want to have reconstructive surgery to replicate your breast, or whether you want to wear a prosthesis in your bra. Consider both the logistical and practical factors as well as the psychological impact. Some women opt for reconstructive surgery to regain a feeling of "wholeness" and maintain a positive body image. Others don't want to endure the extensive, multiple surgical procedures and risks that reconstruction involves over a year or more, or just can't be "bothered" with it all and feel fine about missing a breast. And some are so overwhelmed that they can make only one decision at a time, so they'll opt for mastectomy now, use a prosthesis in the interim, and save the reconstruction decision for later, when they may have more time and perspective to make an informed decision.

There is no "right" answer, only an answer for you. (And don't let your doctors persuade you to reconstruct. In their earnestness to help they often assume that every woman would choose to re-create her breast if possible.) If you do decide to reconstruct, you also need to decide whether to do "immediate reconstruction," in which the first phase of reconstruction is done by the plastic surgeon during the mastectomy operation itself, or whether you want to "delay reconstruction" until you have completed all your treatments and you are better able to cope with it, both physically and emotionally, at some time in the future. Many women point to several advantages of immediate reconstruction: (a) a separate surgery later is eliminated, (b) the patient awakens from surgery with a newly reconstructed breast "mound," which can soften the harsh psychological blow of mastectomy, and (c) the cosmetic results may be enhanced because the surgeon and plastic surgeon are working as a team, rather than sequentially. However, your surgeon will best be able to tell you whether you are a candidate for such procedures.

Phase 2. To Implant or Borrow?

If you choose reconstructive surgery, the next decision is the composition of your new breast. Some women prefer saline implants because they don't want to endure the extensive surgeries and bodily scarring associated with creating a breast mound by moving, or borrowing, your own muscle and tissue from elsewhere on your body. Also, some women's anatomy doesn't permit natural reconstruction, as the surgeon doesn't feel there is sufficient fat or muscle in the back or abdomen, from which tissue is usually taken to recreate a breast. Other women fear anything artificial inserted permanently into their bodies, like saline implants, and view the more extensive surgery of natural reconstruction as the better alternative. Furthermore, while implants may need to be replaced every fifteen years or so, natural reconstruction lasts forever.

Phase 3. Reconstructing the Natural Way: From the Front or Back?

And finally, if you choose your own tissue for reconstruction, your surgeon will discuss with you which method would work best with your body type and anatomy. While both are physically more daunting than many women foresee, the more prevalent method today is the "TRAM Flap" reconstruction, in which tissue is removed from the abdomen, so you have the concurrent benefit of a "tummy tuck" as well. Another choice is the "LAT Flap," where the latissimus dorsi muscle is taken from the upper back and pulled through the underarm to the front of the body to make a breast mound. However, many women don't have enough tissue there for a successful outcome.

This decision framework is admittedly a very cursory overview, but provides the basic road map for consultations with surgeons and plastic surgeons. Of all the decisions you need to make through this whole experience, the mastectomy issues are perhaps the most active, the most personal, and the most complex for you. After all, together with your surgeon, you will decide how to rebuild your body or not.

So If I Have a Choice, Isn't One Even a Teeny Bit Better Than the Other?

Sorry, it's not that easy. If you are given a choice, and the NCI has proven that mastectomy and lumpectomy plus radiation are equivalent in survival rates, then how do you decide which type of surgery is best for you? The "better" option will be your own very personal decision based on a variety of physical and emotional factors, which might include, among other determinants:

- *Recurrence prevention.* First and foremost, which offers your best defense against a recurrence given your particular situation? What do you feel most comfortable with, both physically and emotionally?
- *Body image.* To what extent are your breasts a significant part of your overall body image? Do you feel good about your overall appearance? What role does your chest play in your overall "packaging"?

- *Feminine identity.* To what extent is your breast a symbol of your femininity and sexuality? Do you feel that you would be any less of a woman, or any less attractive, if you were missing a breast?
- *Cosmetic results.* Which alternative provides the best cosmetic result? Would a lumpectomy leave you "uneven"? Would a mastectomy be able to make you appear more "balanced" (either with reconstruction or prosthesis)?
- *Physical tolerance for recovery and rehabilitation.* Since mastectomy is more extensive surgery, how much tolerance do you have for greater physical discomfort and recovery time?
- *Attitude toward reconstructive surgery.* With a mastectomy, are you willing to undergo a series of reconstructive procedures to get the best cosmetic results? Are you willing to live with artificial materials (e.g., saline) in your body forever? Alternatively, are you willing to have muscle and tissue surgically moved from another part of your body to build a new breast? Will your body structure successfully allow for it?
- *Attitude toward radiation.* Since radiation is always part of the lumpectomy treatment and is not necessarily associated with mastectomy, are you willing to go through radiation? Is this a more frightening alternative than the more extensive mastectomy surgery?

And If You Opt Out, a Prosthesis Is Always an Option . . . but Make Sure to Make It Part of Who You Are.

If you have a mastectomy and decide that reconstructive surgery is more than you'd like to endure (at least for now, since you can always reconsider later), then wearing a prosthesis is a very feasible, simple alternative. In addition to the emotional aspects—maintaining a positive body image and your sense of femininity and sensuality, there are also many practical reasons to be well fitted with a prosthesis. If you are moderate- or large-busted, a prosthesis not only will help clothes drape better on your body, but will provide anatomical balance, so your skeletal system (e.g., neck, shoulders, and back) doesn't become misaligned, causing you chronic problems down the road.

About four to six weeks after surgery, you should be healed

enough to be fitted well for a prosthesis. If you try before, you may still be too swollen to get a proper fit. Ask your surgeon, a social worker at the hospital, or other survivors you know to refer you to a prosthesis fitter. This may be at a specialty boutique (generally only if you live in a larger city), a store within the hospital, or even the lingerie section of department stores. Each Nordstrom department store has a prosthesis specialist in every region of the country.

Once you have a list in hand, you might remember the following to make the whole experience a bit less overwhelming (after all, you are being fitted for a whole new body part):

- *Consider the environment impact.* Since this experience is fraught with emotion, some women may prefer to travel a bit farther to a specialty boutique that can handle all their needs (e.g., prostheses, bras, swimsuits, nightwear), and provides a comforting, private, relaxing environment. Others may live near a Nordstrom or other department store which has a "prosthesis coordinator" who can be consulted as a specialist, and which also trains salespeople to be knowledgeable about addressing all the needs of breast cancer survivors, so prosthesis fittings can be integrated into a regular shopping routine. (For more on the Nordstrom program, call 1-800-695-8000 or access their Web site at *www.nordstrom.com*). Decide what works best for you, not only logistically, but emotionally as well.
- *Fit the bra first.* Since the majority of women are walking around wearing the wrong bra size, a benefit you'll get out of this experience is that you'll be properly fitted with the right size for you. If you fit the bra well first, identifying the right size prosthesis is much easier (note there are many standard sizes and shapes to choose from).
- *Any bra can be fitted.* If you don't want to give up some of your favorite bras, bring them in to your prosthesis fitter. Often they can add a lining, or pocket, to your bra, in which the prosthesis can sit comfortably.
- *Your insurance coverage should provide a sufficient wardrobe.* Insurance coverage will vary, but at a minimum, you should be able to get your basic needs covered. For example, Medicare covers one regular prosthesis form, one "lightweight"

form (e.g., for swimming or sports), and four surgical bras per year. Check your policy before you go for your fitting.

- *Make it part of who you are.* Last, and perhaps most important, embrace the prosthesis as part of your body—how you move, who you are. Many women find that as they gain greater emotional comfort with their prosthesis, any physical discomfort they had tended to subside. Learn to accept it and live with it.

Most often, you will walk out of the store completely outfitted after just one visit that takes about an hour. No special orders, no complications, no follow-up surgeries. And maintenance is simple. Since most prostheses today are made of a polyurethane exterior with a silicone interior, you can wash it with soap and water, just like your body. But unlike your body, you have to replace it about every three to four years. It's so easy, it's no wonder why many women opt to avoid reconstructive surgery.

If I Can't Decide, Can I Let Someone Else Make the Decision for Me?

Very definitely, no! While you might be influenced by others and their feelings—your spouse, lover, family, friends—don't let them make the decision for you. Only you, in conjunction with your doctors, can make the choice. It's your body and you have to live with it every day. Eventually, they will get over any fears or anxieties they have regarding your choice, and remember that they love you for who you are, not for the physical package in which you come wrapped. Plus, you don't want to resent someone else forever, if later you decide that you would have chosen a different option. And finally, if the physical structure of your breast significantly affects the nature of an intimate relationship, then it's time for you to re-examine that relationship.

FINANCIAL AND INSURANCE IMPLICATIONS: NOT WHAT YOU NEED RIGHT NOW

Until now, you've probably been overwhelmed and busy just trying to understand your diagnosis, hold yourself together emotionally, get your health care team assembled, and evaluate your treatment options. The last thing you need is insurance or financial hassles. So, before you undergo any type of surgery, you'll need to get savvy about your current coverage and any requirements you need to fulfill to maximize your coverage. Just like the section called "Information Gathering" in Chapter 2, this may be a section you return to repeatedly.

First, Read the Employee Benefits Manual.

It seems pretty obvious, but the very first action you should take in assessing the financial and insurance implications of your diagnosis is probably sitting right in your desk drawer (or your significant other's if you don't work and depend on his health plan for coverage). Stories abound of women who end up in trouble, or get less than optimal coverage, because they simply didn't read their benefits manual to understand the details of the policy. Most people don't pay any attention to this while they are healthy. But it becomes critically important when you need to call on it.

You should be perfectly clear about what you are entitled to, when, with what required notification to whom, and under what conditions. If you are not, make a date with a benefits expert in the human resources department to review it in detail. Only when you fully understand both your health insurance and disability coverage are you ready to talk with your insurance company.

If you still are looking for more information on insurance after talking with your HR department, contact the National Coalition for Cancer Survivorship. (See Chapter 2, "Gathering Information.") Request their publication entitled "What Cancer Survivors Need to Know About Health Insurance," which provides helpful information on the implications for cancer associated with a variety of insurance plans, including fee-for-service, HMO/PPO/POS managed care plans, Medicare, and Medicaid.

Next, Befriend the Insurance Claims Agent (or Management), by Name, Date, Diagnosis Code, Procedure Code, and Confirmation Number.

Get in the practice of recording all names, dates, and direct phone numbers of anyone you talk with from your insurance company. Optimally, you'll want to find a regular contact at your insurer, someone who gets to know your situation. If you get unsatisfactory or vague answers from customer service representatives, move up the organization into higher levels of management until you get satisfactory information. Ask for the individual with overall responsibility for managing your corporation's plan. Be persistent about asking for coverage.

Once you have an individual contact with whom you feel you can develop a good working relationship, make things easier by having all the details of your coverage requests handy, including the diagnosis code and procedure codes (which your doctor provides). Then, whenever you get any information or promises about coverage over the phone, request them in writing to protect yourself should you ever be challenged. Particularly for surgery, get a letter from your insurance company stating their intent to cover the surgical procedures and hospital stay, including the diagnosis code and any procedure codes (sometimes your surgeon's staff will do this for you, but you'll just want to be sure).

Then, Make a Checklist: Your Needs versus Your Insurer's Coverage.

Make a complete list of all the costs you foresee, and the requirements for getting coverage according to your understanding of your health plan. Include costs that you aren't sure about (e.g., wigs, home health care, transportation to and from treatment). At least you can ask about coverage, and if it's denied, you can revise your own monthly budget accordingly. The never-ending list of costs might include:

- Initial consultations, second opinions, and other advice beyond second opinions.
- All surgical procedures, from removal of cancer through recon-

structive phases, if needed (reauthorization is often required for full coverage in a nonemergency situation).

- Deductibles and copayments for each procedure, office visit, treatment.
- Out-of-pocket maximums per year (this is a mixed blessing as the cancer experience will probably bring you to your maximum, but after you hit that threshold, you generally aren't responsible for further payment to your health care providers).
- Coverage for experimental treatments (if you are part of a clinical trial, costs are typically covered by the sponsoring institution—just make sure the costs of remedying unforseen side effects from variations in protocol administration are covered).
- Coverage for any required devices or prostheses, from wigs to breast forms (should you have a mastectomy and decide against reconstruction), including maintenance and upkeep.
- Personal costs, such as transportation to the hospital and treatment center and personal items to make your hospital stay more pleasant.

Armed with an estimate of all the types of costs you are facing, you will be able to plan a budget. Work with your doctors to set up long-term payment plans. We have all been so brainwashed by the media about how the medical community is greedy and arrogant that we forget that most doctors are reasonable, caring, honest people (that's why they're your doctors). Determine how much you can afford each month and offer to pay it until your balance is zero. Your conscientiousness will give you peace of mind that the financial aspects of breast cancer can all be worked out over time.

Establish a Bill-Tracking System.

Prepare yourself for the inundation of medical bills by setting up a system for tracking all these costs. Make it part of your health care "log book" (see Chapter 2, "Building Your Health Care Team"). Whether it's a simple notebook or a more elaborate computer spreadsheet, you need to track each bill at three stages: (a) date of services rendered, (b) date bill was submitted to insurer, by you or directly by the provider, and (c) date payment was received, whether by the provider or by you. For each bill, make sure you also have an itemization of services rendered with the diagnosis codes. Then at the end of each month, review all statements to confirm that your bills are moving through the payment process. If not, it will be your responsibility to call either your doctor's office or the insurance company to resolve any delays or oversights.

If this all seems overwhelming and exhausting, and you just don't have the energy to manage any insurance hassles, ask your spouse, a family member, or someone from your inner circle to help in tracking bills. Just make sure this person can balance his or her own checkbook!

Don't Let Your Insurance Company Dictate What's Best for Your Body: Let Your Health Care Team Go to Bat for What You Need.

In the end, your financial coverage should not drive the decision about what is best for you and your body. We've made much progress, even in the past ten years, improving coverage for the entire range of breast cancer treatments. Today, most surgeries, procedures, and treatments should be covered in the adjuvant setting. Even full coverage for all aspects of mastectomy, including reconstruction, has recently been guaranteed by the Women's Health and Cancer Rights Act of 1998. Sometimes you may still be refuted. Don't give up, as you have several options. Ask your doctor to send a letter to your insurer explaining the medical need for the procedure. Work with his or her administrative staff to do this—remember, you want your doctor to focus on *treating* you, not fighting administrative headaches. You might even ask them to involve their billing service—if they use one—since these organizations deal with health care claims daily, and know how to best work the system. Also, some hospitals have patient representatives, as part of either their billing department or their social work services. These representatives act as advocates for you, negotiating with your insurance company. Hopefully, considering your specific situation will transform you in the eyes of your insurer from an anonymous claim number to a human needing medical care.

If your doctors go to bat for you but you still encounter obstacles, you can ask your doctor to contact his or her state medical society, which can provide you with information on how other similar cases have been resolved. You may uncover more ammunition for your payment argument.

Don't Make Any Drastic Moves Right Now. It Could Be Much More Costly Than Any Treatment Program.

Above all, don't shop for new insurance right now. Stay put! Horror stories abound of women who take dramatic steps upon learning of their diagnosis. Fearing that cancer will cost them dearly, they seek out new, less expensive insurance coverage. Don't even bother looking. Independent insurance is nearly impossible to get postdiagnosis. Before you make any changes, consider both the short- and long-term implications of all alternatives. And don't ever believe a salesman who claims, "Oh, they'll never know about your cancer if you just don't tell them." Wrong! It's not only immoral and unethical, but also untrue.

And If You Still Need Help, Call Lifewise.

If, after you fully explore your insurance coverage and policies, you are still concerned about the financial burden that your cancer experience may impose, you might want to contact Lifewise Family Financial Security. Lifewise, a fully regulated private financial institution, is a highly specialized provider of credit for individuals and families facing life-threatening illnesses (e.g., cancer, heart failure). You can contact them at 1-800-219-7385. At the very least, you might obtain a free copy of their 40-page resource guide that contains an overview of various financial resources for those facing life-theatening illnesses. Additionally, during normal business hours, a staff of oncology nurses is available to answer all types of medical, financial, and insurance questions.

CHAPTER 4
Undergoing Surgery

Much of this chapter discusses routine procedures that might be relevant for any hospital visit, so if you've spent time around hospitals, you might find this section fairly basic. Since I had never been a patient in a hospital before, I found the entire experience a bit overwhelming and intimidating, and as cold and impersonal as those concrete hospital floors you never want to touch without your slippers on. I felt like a registration number that was being moved through an assembly line. So, if you're in my shoes (or slippers), you might just find some of the following advice alleviates that pre-hospital anxiety and makes the actual hospital stay a bit more palatable and comfortable.

THE HOSPITAL VISIT

Presurgery Testing: Just One More Test?

About a week prior to surgery, you'll be asked to go to the hospital for preadmission testing; this is mandatory for anyone requiring a surgical procedure under general anesthesia. And no, it's not just one test, but several, including blood work, a chest X ray, an EKG (which monitors your heart rate), and possibly others. In some cases, your general internist will do this at his or her office. At this time, make sure you notify the medical professionals of any allergies you have or any medications you're on (they will surely ask you this), as they should know if you need to be weaned off any medications that might interfere with your surgery or anesthesia. Plan to devote at least an entire morning or afternoon to this process. And bring someone with you, partially to pass the time, and partially to distract you from worrying about what's still to come. Otherwise, your mind may terrorize you before you even leave the waiting room!

The Night Before . . . Pronounce a Fond Farewell . . .

You won't believe it until you are forced to encounter it, and it may sound downright silly, but many women who have undergone mastectomies created their own very private rituals to say good-bye to their breast. Several women I've spoken with mentioned a long, calming soak in a bathtub. Some created visualizations or meditations on their "new" bodies. Some made love. And one woman even had her chest photographed portrait-style to immortalize her original body. They each needed to grieve and mourn the process in anticipation of the reality. And those women to whom it didn't occur to create a ritual frequently voiced regret that they hadn't had such foresight and creativity.

Schedule Surgery in the Morning. Prevent Both Panic and Big Mac Attacks.

If at all possible, try to have your surgery scheduled for the morning. First, you won't have to spend the better part of the day anxious and nervous about going into surgery (you probably won't sleep much the night before anyway, so why not just get on with it). And second, you won't be allowed to eat or drink anything after midnight the day before, so morning surgery eliminates excessive hunger or thirst.

Bring Reading Material (Preferably Post-1993) . . .

Just because your surgery is scheduled for a particular time, don't expect to be whisked away at the exact moment. In fact, expect to wait, and wait, and wait. At first, you'll wait with your family members or friends who accompany you to the hospital. After a while, however, you'll be taken alone to a preop waiting room, which feels like a holding tank. There may be some medical staff to talk with and distract you, but your surest bet is to bring some reading material that you can become absorbed in. Since I hadn't brought anything with me, my only entertainment for more than an hour was some old magazines scattered around the waiting room . . . from 1993! I forced myself to read them—anything was better than dwelling on surgery. But a great novel or juicy magazine would have been a much better alternative!

. . . Unless, of Course, You Can't See Anyway.

If you wear glasses or contact lenses, be prepared to be in a fog—literally and figuratively—for that period before surgery. You'll be asked to leave any eyewear in the changing room with your clothes, so if your eyesight isn't great, make sure the nurse escorts you wherever you need to go. And make sure your reading material has large-enough type or you have plenty of light!

A Day in the Life of a Lumpectomy . . .

If you are undergoing a lumpectomy, you'll be sent home from the hospital before the flowers from well-wishers start wilting. Generally, you are in and out within about twenty-four hours, with a recent trend to same-day outpatient surgery due to advances in surgical techniques. The actual procedure takes two to three hours, including the lymph node dissection. After time in the recovery room, and the stabilization of your vital signs, you may be moved to a room, but only if you are to spend the night. The next day the nurses will have you walking around—albeit slowly and perhaps in some pain—and by the end of the day you'll be on your way home. It's such a short hospital stay, you might ask your visitors to greet you at home.

. . . And a Few Days in the Life of a Mastectomy (with some Follow-Up Visits).

The more extensive surgery associated with a mastectomy requires a longer hospital stay, generally ranging from two to six days. The surgery itself may last up to six to seven hours if your plastic surgeon teams with your general surgeon to begin the reconstruction process. Many women report that upon waking, and for the next several days, they are surprised at how battered and sore they feel across their entire body. They feel as if they've been hit by a Mack truck. And what they all began to realize is just how many muscle groups are connected to and interact with the chest and arm muscles. Almost everything across your trunk is interconnected. So, what were some of their favorite remedies (to supplement, not replace, the painkillers)? One clever woman I spoke with arranged to have her masseuse come to the hospital several times to do some gentle bodywork. Other solutions included: bringing a favorite soft blanket or comforter from home, building stacks of pillows to prop up your arm and trunk, asking the nurses for extra help to sit up and move, or even listening to relaxation or visualization tapes to calm and soothe the muscles. If you are so inclined and can afford it, you might consider hiring a private nurse for the initial day or two.

Besides finding ways to increase physical comfort, the other major challenge seems to be managing the flow of visitors and well-wishers. Remember that you're entitled to be a bit self-indulgent right now. If you're too exhausted for visitors, ask them to come another day, or call to see when you might be feeling stronger and more prepared for company.

P.S. If you have chosen any type of breast reconstruction, you will require a series of follow-up surgeries, from insertion of tissue expanders for implants, to creating a new nipple, either by skin graft or tattoo. Ask your surgeon to map out a schedule for the entire series of procedures. However, don't get too attached to any formal "completion date" as there are often setbacks or delays based on your body's own healing process.

Relax. Surgery Is the Easy Part. (Sorry!)

In retrospect, I think that actually undergoing the surgery is the easiest part of this ordeal. Why? Maybe it's because I'm a very practical and results-focused person, but I was comforted by the fact that:

- *It's easily comprehended.* There's a physical lump which the surgeon removes.

- *It's decisive.* Surgery hopefully removes the cancer from your body, forever, end of discussion, that's it, no more.
- *There are tangible results.* Your scars heal, you regain your arm mobility, you recover from surgery, and you feel good.
- *There's closure.* You know when it's over, and you know if the tumor was completely removed. Convince yourself that surgery is not really that bad, that it will be over soon, and that you'll be fine. Save your mental fortitude for the more complicated decisions around treatment alternatives, and the endurance to get through those seemingly endless months of treatment.

Make Sure You're Not Going "Home Alone."

When it comes time to leave the hospital, make sure you have someone to: (a) take you home from the hospital, and (b) stay with you for the first three to four days. Why?

- *First, the pain and limited mobility.* Sorry for reminding you. Whether you underwent a lumpectomy or a mastectomy, you may be in a fair amount of pain. (Don't ever refuse a pain-killer; that's what they're made for, and there's nothing heroic or beneficial in abstaining!) Plus, you won't have enough arm and shoulder mobility to open your car door, let alone drive yourself home.
- *Second, you can never predict the aftereffects of anesthesia.* You could be groggy and/or nauseous for several days, not to mention that your painkillers may knock you out as well.
- *Third, the drain.* While the hospital staff will try to educate you about the drain that will be inserted into your lymph node area during surgery, you won't fully realize how awkward it is until after you're completely awake again. It looks and works like a turkey baster inserted in your underarm. For five to ten days, depending on your body and how it heals, this drain will capture excess fluids which tend to build up in this area. You may need to have someone empty and clean it if you can't reach it or you are not yet emotionally ready to look at your surgery area.

Make sure that whoever stays with you is someone who can also be supportive and encouraging at this time (and not to mention, doesn't faint at the sight of blood). If you don't want to be a "burden" on anyone for too long because your friends and family have other obligations besides devoting themselves to you for several days, try rotating. I had one relative with me through surgery and going home, another for two days thereafter, and a friend who then came for the weekend.

If for any reason you don't have someone to bring you home, talk to a nurse or a social worker at your hospital, or call your local American Cancer Society to inquire about a home health aide or visiting nurse. There's always someone willing to help, so don't be afraid to ask for it. Your insurance may cover this service.

CHAPTER 5
Recovering from Surgery

Recovering from surgery is a fine balance. On the one hand, you need to allow yourself to be pampered a bit, to save your strength for the healing process. On the other hand, you want to set goals for yourself fairly early on as a means to get yourself on the road to recovery. The sooner you start, the quicker your recovery. However, be patient, as the healing process varies tremendously according to a multitude of factors. This chapter will cover:

- *Recovering from Surgery*, including both helpful hints on the physical aspects of healing as well as some of the emotional aftermath to be prepared for.
- Some of the *Long-term Implications* and daily reminders that you may need to learn to live with (remember, though, you're happy just to be alive).
- The meaning of the additional information gleaned from your *Surgery Results* in your pathology report, which your health care team will use to make the optimal treatment recommendation for you.

THE QUICK ROAD TO RECOVERY

First, Pamper Yourself. Then Set Goals and Reach Milestones.

I can't emphasize enough that this is the one time in your life that you should let others care for you and do things for you, without feeling an obligation to return the favor. Let yourself be pampered and cared for by anyone and everyone. Savor it. Also, do things for yourself that make you feel good. Get massages; get a makeover (perhaps from the Look Good, Feel Better® program of the ACS). Women who have been through mastectomies mentioned that buying new sexy lingerie helped them get over the loss of their breast. However, you need to temper the luxury of pampering with the reality of setting goals for yourself and returning to the activities of life.

While I established mostly physical exercise goals for myself, some women aspired to milestone events, however large or small. One woman simply wanted to be able to attend the opera several weeks after her surgery, to maintain her regular season series. Another wanted to dance at her son's wedding the next month in a pretty new dress. It doesn't matter what it is. Just have a milestone, a light at the end of your tunnel.

So When Is Everyone Going to Stop Telling Me I'm Courageous, and Just Admit They Feel Sorry for Me?

I suppose it's a wonderful compliment in very strange packaging, but upon my return to work after surgery, I was soon ready to punch the next person who told me how much he or she admired my strength, and how courageously I was handling my cancer diagnosis. Yeah, right! I guess they couldn't imagine the number of moments I was so terrified that I felt like a deer frozen in a car's headlights. Okay, it's nice to receive words of encouragement and praise about courage, but it would also be nice just to get a big hug (but don't squeeze too hard, because that would really hurt just now) and have someone say, "I feel terrible for you, honey, and while I can't even begin to understand what you're going through, I'll be here for anything you need." Enough of the admiration . . . pamper me!

Involve Your Partner Early and Often.

One of the most uncomfortable aspects of healing from surgery can be the worry about how your spouse or significant other will deal with your bodily changes. If you start with the premise that a good relationship should withstand a mastectomy, then your partner should be intimately involved from the start. In fact, the earlier he or she is involved in physically caring for you, the better your partner may be at coping with your loss; and the less uncomfortable you'll feel, with no official "unveiling" hanging over your head. Asking your partner to help change your drain, or to be with you the first time your bandages are changed, removes the entire situation from the more emotionally charged sexual context to one of simply helping an individual heal from a wound. Then, once you are physically feeling stronger, you can ease back into the sexual relationship with which both of you are comfortable.

About This Drain . . . Consider It Your Newfound Friend.

The drain might repel you because it's a constant reminder of your recent surgery or because you just don't fare well at the sight of blood. Alternatively, you can also view it as your newfound friend, as a measure of your progress in healing. Each day when you (or your caretaker or partner) empties it, you measure the amount of fluid, which decreases over time. When it's low enough, your surgeon removes it by simply pulling it out during a visit to his or her office. Now you can really be on the road to recovery, since it will get easier and easier to move your arm and shoulder.

Try Arnica Oil to Avoid Feeling like a Balloon.

Arnica oil is a homeopathic remedy that can help mitigate post-surgical swelling. The arnica plant is often mixed with oils and even fragrances and sold as a massage oil, but the more ingredients, the less pure, so look for a brand that is composed simply of arnica extract and olive oil. You may find it at your local health food store. Just rub it gently on the chest area, avoiding the actual incision site.

There's More Than One Way to Mend a Seam . . . or Heal a Scar.

Regardless of the extent of physical changes to your chest, you'll be worried about scars on your formerly flawless body (don't we all wish!). A few remedies that women have sworn by include: vitamin E oil or capsules, calendula cream, cocoa butter, and even raw aloe directly from the plant (beware the prepackaged gel, as it contains alcohol that can be drying and irritating). Wait until your wounds are completely closed up, and your stitches have been removed. Then, applying any of these once or twice a day (all should be available at your local health food store) will help keep the skin soft and pliable, so the scars are minimized in both redness and texture. Finally, there's a variety of new products on the market, such as Cica-Care or Rejuveness, that are somewhat pricey fabric-type "patches" that you cut to the shape of your scar. Over several days of repeated application, the medicine in the fabric fades your scars. Sounds like a miracle cure? Maybe, but ask your doctor before rushing to your nearest medical supply store, as he or she will probably have an opinion as to which might be most effective.

Consider Your Scars Medals of Honor.

Knowing that the word "scar" means permanent marking, and that your scars will never disappear completely, consider your scars medals of honor for a battle you so valiantly fought and won! As one woman exclaimed to me, "I love my scars. They saved my life!"

The Surgical Bra: Not Exactly a Candidate for the Next Victoria's Secret Catalog Cover.

You may awaken from surgery wearing a "surgical bra" which will be yours to keep. Lucky you! You probably haven't seen something like this since you gave up your training bras in your preadolescent days. As a soft cotton bra with a front Velcro closure, they aren't exactly sexy, but they are the most comfortable and convenient garments you can wear for the next few weeks (until your surgeon gives you the okay to return to the world of regular undergarments), and they will hold you in place to avoid any pain associated with extra movement. Just make sure you wear dark-colored shirts to hide their slight bulkiness. Or wear a thin white cotton T-shirt or camisole over your surgical bra to prevent any strange lines from screaming out from under your shirt.

Note that there may be other variations of bandaging and dressing for mastectomy patients, but the advice about cotton shirts and dark colors is still very apropos.

Next, Rotate Your Bras for Greater Comfort (and Make the Lingerie Department of Your Local Store Very Happy).

Once you've graduated from the surgical bra, you might return to your old bras only to find that they should be sent directly to the trash bin. Depending on the invasiveness of your surgery and the location of your incisions, you may not be able to wear the styles you had previously, particularly underwires, at least until complete healing has occurred, which can take a year or more. So, what to do? Go to your nearest department store, as they typically have the most varied selection of bra styles. Buy yourself several different styles of soft cotton or mesh bras. If you rotate the styles each day, you won't irritate any one particular spot on your chest. Plus, you'll be in the height of fashion with your new undergarment wardrobe. Walk through any lingerie department and see all the mannequins adorned in the unstructured, camisole-style bras.

Make Dates with Yourself or Take Up New Activities, Just to Prove You're in Working Order.

One of the hardest emotional aspects of surgery for me was convincing myself during the recuperation phase that I would be restored to "normal" working order, and that I would have full range of motion in my arm and shoulder. So, what to do? I made a date with myself to prove that I'd be fine. Just twenty days after my surgery, I went to play tennis. No, I did not play a full three sets and beat my opponent. In fact, I hit for only twenty minutes, and couldn't even lift my arm above my head well enough to serve. But all that was important was that I did it. I was out there on the tennis court, swinging my racquet just like normal (okay, a bit slower and softer), and everything worked. It reinforced my belief that my body would return to "normal." It was a terrific emotional triumph. Another woman I spoke with took up fly fishing in her postmastectomy days. Not only did she find it relaxing and peaceful (back to that nature theme for coping), but it involved extensive arm movement, so it was great rehabilitation exercise!

Nobody Has a Perfect Pair.

You probably never walked around assessing other women's chests before your surgery. Now you do. Remember, if breast cancer is a one-in-eight phenomenon, there are at least a few other women on your daily commute to work, school, wherever, who have had some type of surgery. And furthermore, Mother Nature never really gets them quite even. So, instead of being timid or embarrassed that you might be scarred or a bit lopsided, flaunt them. As one double-mastectomy survivor declared to me, "If people can parade around in $60,000 BMWs, why can't I parade my $60,000 chest?"

The World Won't Be Staring at Your Chest. Or Maybe They Will.

One of the universal but strange emotional aftermaths of surgery is an incredible feeling of exposure and vulnerability. Regardless of whether you had a lumpectomy or mastectomy, you venture out into the world convinced that not a person will pass you without staring at your chest, transparent for all to see. Calm your imagination and paranoia. Not everyone is staring . . . and even if they are, perhaps it's due to your new and improved version.

Body Image: A Strange Whirlwind of Emotions (and Yes, You Might Even Feel Sexier).

You've just undergone major surgery that may have significantly altered your body shape, and should have damaged your body image and self-esteem. However, paradoxically many women find that they feel stronger and more confident than ever from overcoming the challenges of surgery. You realize that you're still the same person, regardless of your altered figure, with the same feelings, attitudes, and perspectives on life. Just because your body has changed doesn't mean you've changed (you've only become stronger)! This knowledge and insight can be very empowering and liberating. Your newfound strength may be so contagious and radiant that you exude a certain sexiness you never knew you had.

Exercise: Just (Try to) Do It.

No, I'm not the advertising director for Nike, but I am a passionate advocate of exercise as part of a lifelong health program (you'll hear more later). All the hype you've ever heard about the benefits of exercise—from doctors, from the media, from any sports coaches/trainers you might have had—is true, and now more than ever. Although your Number One task right now is to recover from your surgery, and it will require a lot of your body's energy to do that, any exercise program that you can maintain, even if scaled back quite substantially, will provide the following benefits:

- *Strengthen your immune system.* One of the main benefits of aerobic exercise, even 20–30 minutes, 3–4 times per week, is a stronger immune system. If you are following surgery with chemotherapy, you'll want your immune system as strong as possible as you head into treatment since chemo may weaken your immune system.
- *Maintain physical stamina and strength.* Since people in good, strong physical condition tend to tolerate chemotherapy better than those who are weaker[1], try to keep yourself as strong as possible. Look at it this way: Chemo can make you weak and take a lot out of you; the higher your level of physical conditioning, the higher your "low" will be. I found it impossible to maintain my regular workout at the gym (I was far too weak, tired, and in pain), but I did try to either walk 1–2 miles or ride my bike 5–6 miles at a leisurely pace, almost every day. I never exerted myself too much to put undue stress on my body, but I felt that I was at least keeping the blood flowing and the muscles working.
- *Facilitate a quicker physical recovery.* While surgery, and

1. *I Can Cope: Staying Healthy with Cancer,* Judi Johnson and Linda Klein, CHRONIMED Publishing, 1994, p. 49.

subsequent treatments, can damage muscle and tissue, exercise can help rebuild the damaged cells by increasing the blood flow to the damaged area.

- *Provide peace of mind.* Needless to say, the entire surgery ordeal is filled with anxiety and uncertainty, so maintaining your exercise program as much as possible is a tremendous emotional outlet, both in terms of stress relief and the feeling that you are keeping your life as normal as possible during this time, and do have some control over it.

At the bare minimum, just try to walk a mile or so every day. Of course, check with your doctor before beginning or continuing any exercise regimen during this time. (For more on the importance of an ongoing exercise program, see Chapter 8, "Transitioning Back to 'Normal.' ")

And Add a Special Program for Your Shoulder, Arm, and Chest.

Regardless of whether you had a lumpectomy or a mastectomy, most doctors today agree that the sooner you get your arm and shoulder moving, the better. Most likely, your surgeon, nurses, and/or physical therapists will give you a series of arm exercises to restore the full range of motion and flexibility you had prior to surgery. Among others, specific exercises might include[2]:

- *Pendulum*—Swing your arm from left to right while bent forward at the waist to loosen your shoulder.
- *Exaggerated deep breathing*—Inhale deeply and slowly to expand your chest muscles.
- *Clasp-lift-stretch*—Clasp your hands together on your lap, and slowly raise them above your forehead, keeping elbows in.
- *Back climb*—Clasp your hands behind your back and slowly slide them up to the middle of your back.
- *Wall climb*—Standing facing a wall, "crawl" your arms progressively higher up the wall, with your elbows straight, and moving your body closer to the wall over time.

2. "Arm Exercises: A Program After Breast Surgery," from the Strang-Cornell Breast Center, New York, New York.

In addition, use everyday chores and tasks to help yourself as well. Stretch yourself to reach for that object on the top shelf. But don't ever do anything that hurts too much, and stop if your arm is getting tired.

Hesitant about Life and Sports Activities? Okay, but Only with a Little H.

You might find that when you first return to life/athletic activities postsurgery, you're a bit more timid or hesitant than usual. That's okay. You're normal. Although you may have been riding a bike since it had training wheels, you're now completely convinced that the next time you ride downhill, the brakes will lock, you will fly over the handlebars, your skin will become instant sandpaper on the gravel, and lymphedema will plague you forever. It's not likely to happen, but just to make sure, you might think about protecting your arm a bit more on future rides.

LONG-TERM IMPLICATIONS: DAILY REMINDERS

Well after you've healed from surgery, there may be a few lingering physical reminders of the trauma your body has endured. However, with a little awareness and planning, they are all very manageable.

Scar Tissue Can Be Very Misleading. Use a Band-Aid to Trick Yourself.

Scar tissue runs deep. You might have moments of panic as your surgery heals, when you still feel a lump or something hard either directly underneath or in the area around the incision site. Most likely, it is not a cancer recurrence, or a piece of tumor left behind, but simply internal scar tissue. It's not likely to be worrisome. Just leave it alone, so you don't irritate it, but do call it to your doctor's attention on your next office visit. When I did, my doctor instructed me to put a Band-Aid over the site, because then I would leave it alone and not rub it obsessively to make sure it was going away.

Your Underarm Nerves Might Only Be Injured, Not Dead. Be Careful If You're Ticklish.

After surgery you may have some loss of feeling in your armpit and inner upper arm area. Sensory nerves were severed during the surgery to remove your lymph node sample. However, don't despair. It may take up to a year or more, but eventually you should get some of that feeling back. Nobody can tell you how much will return or how long it will take, but sensation should improve. Only in rare situations is the damage significant enough to impede a "normal" lifestyle (okay, so if you're planning to play Wimbledon next year, you might have a setback here). And if you're ticklish, maybe loss of feeling is good news!

The Aftermath of Lymph Node Removal: Lymphedema and Cellulitis Risk.

Lymphedema is one of those topics that may or may not be discussed in great detail prior to surgery because if you were told the full implications, you might say no to surgery! Under laws of informed consent, you are required to be told, but in a long laundry list of all the surgery issues, it appears as a minor detail, something like, "Oh yes, there's a risk that you might awake from surgery with some swelling, either temporary or permanent." Wait a minute here! Is there nothing I can do? The scariest thing about lymphedema is that nobody can tell you when, where, how, or if it will happen to you, either now, next year, or forever. But up to 20 percent of all women who have lymph node dissections will develop it at some point.

Technically, lymphedema, a chronic swelling of the hand and/or arm, is caused by blockage in the lymph system to the arm. The blockage is usually due to scar tissue from surgery or the less effective drainage your lymph system can muster in the absence of the lymph nodes you had removed. It can also be caused by radiation to the area where your lymph nodes were removed (but this is rarely done today). In addition to swelling, lymph system damage can result in limited mobility and vulnerability to infection, or cellulitis. Even minimal lymphedema can make the arm ripe for infection, and an infection can exacerbate or cause new lymphedema, which can become permanent.

Think of lymphedema and cellulitis as two halves of a vicious circle that you don't want to get caught up in. To avoid them at all costs, pay attention to early warning signs. Call your doctor at the first signs of pain, discomfort, or swelling. You may be referred to a therapist specializing in lymphatic drain massage, who will work with you to minimize swelling. Treated early, both are manageable. Don't leave them untreated, especially an infection, which can get serious, quickly.

Yes, lymphedema can be a constant reminder that your body has been violated. But given the alternative—that you wouldn't know if your cancer had spread beyond your breast—you just learn to live with it, and minimize it, if it actually appears at some point.

Airplanes Might Turn You into an Elephant Lady.

If you fly on a regular basis, you might be told that changes in cabin pressure inside airplanes can trigger lymphedema. Why take the chance? Have your surgeon send you to be fitted for a compression sleeve, a neoprene or elasticized nylon casing that looks almost like an Ace bandage. Slide it on before the plane takes off and wear it for the duration of the flight as a precaution. You'll never have to know if the airplane might trigger it for you. A side benefit: If you're wearing your sleeve with a short-sleeved shirt (say, during the summer), all sorts of people will offer to help you with your baggage when you get off the plane.

If you plan to fly, ask your surgeon for a prescription, and the location of the nearest facility that can fit you appropriately. Part of the fitting process for a compression sleeve is to take measurements of your arm in several different places. These measurements are good to have as a baseline, should you ever need them, to monitor whether your arm has swollen enough to seek out treatment.

A NOTE FROM ALL THE DOCTORS

R̷x   *Ten Ways to Prevent Lymphedema . . .*

While nobody will guarantee you that you can absolutely prevent lymphedema, the best defense is to pamper your arm a bit more than usual, and be extra careful about preventing injury, trauma, infection, or breaks in the skin of the arm. A few ways to do this include:

1. Keep your arm and hand clean and moisturized on a daily basis.
2. Avoid any unnecessary cuts or punctures of the skin, for example, cutting cuticles, drawing blood, receiving intravenous medications in the affected arm.
3. Avoid excessive pressure on the arm, for example, tight-fitting clothes or jewelry, blood pressure monitors, heavy handbags, or shoulder straps.
4. Wear gloves or protective handgear for any activity where the affected hand might be exposed or vulnerable (e.g., gardening, dishwashing, cooking, housecleaning, sewing, sports).
5. Avoid sunburn and tan gradually. Wear sunscreen with at least SPF-15. In fact, avoid all burns.
6. Avoid insect bites. Carry insect repellent with you throughout the summer.
7. Avoid extreme heat or cold, or sudden temperature changes.
8. Avoid salty foods. Salt retains fluid.
9. Avoid lifting or carrying heavy items or lifting weights for prolonged periods.
10. Avoid activities with constant repetition. Give your arm an occasional rest if you can't avoid repetition.

Carry a topical antibiotic ointment (and Band-Aids) with you at all times, and apply immediately if you do get a cut or break in your skin. Despite all these precautions, if you do see swelling or any other sign of an infection appear—pain, redness, heat—call your doctor immediately. An infection can trigger the swelling of lymphedema, as well as get serious on its own very quickly. When in doubt about injury or infection and what should be done, call or see your medical doctor as soon as possible. Early treatment generally averts bigger problems.

More extensive and current information is always available from the National Lymphedema Network by calling 1-800-541-3259 or accessing their Web site at www.lymphnet.org.

... And a Flash of Good News

The medical community has admitted that lymphedema has been understudied and that treatments are not as effective as they could be. In 1998, the American Cancer Society convened a multidisciplinary group, including representatives from the National Lymphedema Network and NABCO as the first step in making a commitment to research targeted at prevention and effective treatment interventions.

SURGERY RESULTS: ADDING TO THE INFORMATION BASE

Demystifying the Language of Pathology . . . A Road Map Back to Health (but Not without a Lot of Anxiety).

Following surgery, your tumor, any surrounding tissue removed, and the lymph node sampling removed will be sent to a pathologist, who will conduct a battery of laboratory tests on the cancer cells. Pathologists are doctors who specialize in the identification, analysis, and behavior of cells. The test results are summarized in a pathology report, which serves as the basis for your surgeon and oncologists to make follow-up treatment decisions. It's essentially a road map with many signs that indicate the optimal treatment for you to make sure your cancer doesn't return. About a week after surgery, your surgeon will receive your pathology report, and should schedule an appointment to walk you through it. Make sure you have time enough that you fully understand the implications, as they may provide clues to your long-term health.

Warning! Many women have commented that the anxiety and anticipation of receiving pathology results can be overwhelming, perhaps one of the most difficult emotional aspects of the entire experience. Through surgery, I had been pretty much functioning on autopilot, just trying to get through the hospital experience and physical recovery process, and quite frankly, I was in a bit of a fog mentally, not really focusing on anything besides the logistics of surgery. However, the night before going to get my pathology results, I was an absolute mess. The magnitude of what I had just undergone smacked me in the face with a rude awakening . . . *cancer!* I finally comprehended that I had just had cancer surgery, and might be facing my own mortality the very next day. Up to then, I don't think it had ever occurred to me that I might not be alive one, five, or ten years later. Call it denial, call it self-preservation, but my thoughts never entertained the concept of death. But thankfully the results were hopeful and optimistic, as they are for most women with early-stage breast cancer.

To prepare yourself, you might want to be distracted the day before you get your pathology report back. Call on friends and family to help you through this, even if it's as simple as going to a light-hearted movie (no tearjerkers needed today).

A NOTE FROM THE ONCOLOGIST

Breaking the Code: Reading a Pathology Report

Depending on your hospital's pathology department, the types and forms of tests conducted might vary slightly, but there are several standard indicators and commonalities regarding your "prognosis" or potential for long-term survival:

- **Tumor histology.** Histology distinguishes the "type" of breast cancer, of which there are several. The majority of women will be diagnosed with "infiltrating ductal carcinoma," with "infiltrating lobular carcinoma" as the second most common. Sometimes, the histological subtype can have prognostic significance.
- **Lymph node involvement.** The presence of cancer cells that have traveled from the breast into the lymph

nodes is significant, as it may indicate that the cancer has begun to travel to other parts of your body. The absence or presence of cancer in your lymph nodes will help your oncologist determine the most appropriate regimen of chemotherapy. Generally, the more nodes involved, the more aggressive chemotherapy you may receive—both in terms of more toxic drugs and greater duration.

- **Tumor size.** The size of the tumor is very important prognostically, and is measured in centimeters across the widest section of the mass.

- **Tumor grade.** Grade is an assessment of how closely the tumor cells resemble normal breast cells. "Well-differentiated" tumors may look like slightly abnormal breast tissue but maintain the structure of a gland, while "poorly differentiated" tumors look like clusters of round cells that don't resemble normal cell structures. Sometimes, the Bloom-Richardson rating system is used to measure the rate of cell division, differences among cells, and appearance versus normal tissue. Generally, poorly differentiated tumors have a worse prognosis because they're more aggressive.

- **Estrogen and progesterone receptors (ER and PR).** This test indicates whether your cancer cells are "receptive" to, or are fueled by, the two hormones estrogen and/or progesterone. They will be listed as "positive" or "negative" (and may or may not have a specific numeric value as well). Prognostically, positive receptor tumors tend to be less aggressive, so it is better to be positive for both. Additionally, if cells are ER+, the likelihood of response to the drug tamoxifen is higher, so it may be recommended by your oncologist (see Chapter 6, "Tamoxifen, The Hormone Option").

- **HER2-neu.** This is a gene that has prognostic significance, particularly in larger tumors. Tumors that are positive for the HER2-neu gene tend to be more aggressive than those that are negative. However, HER2-neu positive tumors may benefit from Herceptin, an antibody to HER2-neu, so it can be a blessing in disguise! It is generally given for a full year.

- **S-Phase.** As a measurement of the rapidity with which cells are dividing, the S-Phase may be a prognostic indicator, but the clinical debate is ongoing.
- **Oncotype-DX.** Your doctor may wish to order this 21-gene assay performed on the tumor tissue to help determine whether chemotherapy should be given. This is especially helpful in tumors without lymph node involvement that are relatively small.

In general, tumor size and lymph node involvement are the most significant prognostic factors. However, it is also important to realize that only 10 percent of all women will have a pathology report that contains no negative prognostic factors. Therefore, 90 percent will have some type of negative prognostic indicator on their reports. Discuss these with your doctor. Take comfort that your treatment program will address and mitigate these.

Note that many of these prognostic factors tend to "break down" or become less predictive in small tumors—those less than 1 centimeter—because the overriding indicator is that the tumor is so small that the survival prognosis is excellent.

In a Pathology Report, Positive Isn't Necessarily Good.

You always thought that the word "positive" had good connotations? Not necessarily. In breast cancer, it can be either good or bad. If your pathology report indicates "positive lymph node involvement," that's not great, as it means that most likely the cancer cells have started to travel to other parts of your body from your breast through your lymph channels. However, if your cells are "estrogen-positive," that can be good, because you may be a candidate for a hormone therapy treatment like tamoxifen, which is less toxic and grueling than chemotherapy. But if you are in your childbearing years, the downside of being "estrogen-positive" is that it may be riskier to get pregnant since the hormone surges associated with pregnancy may trigger cancer cell growth. So don't rush to make any judgment from the word "positive" (or "negative"). It's all in the context.

Clear Margins Give the Go-Ahead for the Next Phase of Treatment.

If you had a lumpectomy, another piece of information gleaned from your pathology report is whether or not you had "clear" margins around your tumor site. Essentially, your surgeon removes the actual tumor mass with a "healthy" margin of surrounding tissue, just to make sure he or she theoretically "gets" all the cancer cells (and radiation cleans up any that might have "scattered" from the original tumor site). If the entire "halo" of tissue looks healthy under the microscope, you are declared to have "clear" margins, and are able to move on to your next stage of treatment. If, unfortunately, there is cancerous tissue that extends beyond the margins, you have "positive" or "involved" margins, which must be resolved before you can proceed. One option is simply to have the surgeon go back into the original surgical site and "re-excise" more tissue to aim for clear margins. Alternatively, if it seems that the malignant cells are more pervasive throughout the breast tissue, then your health care team may recommend mastectomy.

On This "Stage," You're the Leading Attraction (Unfortunately).

If you're reading this book, you've probably been told you have "early-stage" breast cancer, although you may or may not have been told specifically that you are Stage I or Stage II. All this discussion about "staging" is nothing more than a simple but confusing system for clinically determining the probability that your cancer has spread to other parts of your body. Quite simply, the medical community uses four basic stages to typecast you, based on a "TNM" classification, which stands for: (a) Tumor size, (b) presence or absence of Node involvement, and how many, and (c) whether there is clear evidence of Metastasis. Corresponding to each is a percentage estimate of "survival rates" for five and ten years after your cancer diagnosis. However, there are so many variations on the basic framework and factors specific to your own situation that you need to take the statistics with a grain of salt. I myself found the statistics absolutely terrifying and refused to look at them.

In addition, not once did any of my doctors come out and specif-

ically state, "You have Stage __ cancer." Rather than dwelling on
survival statistics—or mortality, depending on how you look at it—
my doctors kept me focused on the positive by proclaiming, "Your
prognosis is optimistic, as we've caught the cancer in the early
stages." Hopefully, you've heard similar words of encouragement
from your health care team.

For a more clinical discussion of staging, please refer to some of
the references mentioned in Chapter 2, "Gathering Information."

A Second Opinion from a Leading Institution Is Only a FedEx Away.

No matter how comfortable with and confident you are about
your health care team, it is always smart to get a second opinion for
any treatment that potentially can have a lifetime impact. A good
idea is to obtain a review either from one of the country's NCI-
designated comprehensive cancer centers or from a leading university teaching hospital. Just call the pathology department and request an "outside review" of your slides. If you don't live near the
institution that you would like to provide your review, you can simply ask your primary hospital to courier your slides, pathology report, and any other pertinent information. Expect to pay a nominal
charge—not as much as a full in-person consultation—but it should
be covered by your insurance.

Refer back to Chapter 2, "Gathering Information," for more on
resources to guide you and second opinions.

Understand Your Hospital's Archiving Policy. It May Be the Key to Your Future Cure.

Not only is it important to learn the pathology characteristics of
your particular cancer to understand the treatment recommendations, but your pathology report contains valuable information that
may be used in the future to cure you of your specific disease. How?
With continued advances in research and treatments, particularly
in the field of gene therapy, the medical world is getting close to
being able to develop customized treatments specifically for your
cancer cells. Vaccines are one promising area. In the near future,
your oncologist may be able to create a vaccine from pieces of your
original tumor that immunizes your body against its own cancer

cells. So, you want to make sure that the hospital where you had your surgery will store your original tumor slides indefinitely, and if they don't, make sure you request that they are sent to you for keeping at the end of the holding period. This way, should you ever face a recurrence, you will be prepared to take advantage of leading-edge treatments.

A NOTE FROM ALL THE DOCTORS

R̶x Adding Up the Facts: How Doctors Come to a Recommendation

Doctors need to add up all the factors regarding a patient in order to make an informed decision about the appropriate treatment. First, he or she will evaluate the patient's overall state of health. Is she young or older, premenopausal or post-menopausal? Does she have other medical conditions that might interfere with or be affected by treatment options, or is she otherwise healthy? Is she psychologically competent to understand the ramifications and abide by the regimen of treatment? Is she able to appreciate the need for taking some risks in order to improve her chances of survival?

Next, the information gleaned from the pathology report about the actual tumor characteristics must be evaluated. How large is it? Are the estrogen and progesterone receptors positive or negative (i.e., will the tumor respond to hormone therapy)? How aggressive do the cells appear to be under the microscope? How fast are they dividing? What do the other prognostic indicators tell you (see "A Note from the Oncologist: Breaking the Code: Reading a Pathology Report," above)? Is there cancer in the lymph nodes?

After looking at all these factors, the medical oncologist, surgeon, and (if appropriate) radiation oncologist will formulate a recommended treatment for your own specific situation.

Rules of the Road for Family, Friends, and Other Participants

With the surgery phase often comes a sense of urgency, that she must hurry up and do something quickly to get the cancer out of her body. There never seems to be enough time to make some complex decisions about her own body that will have repercussions for the rest of her life. Yet you are all still reeling from the diagnosis. How do you support her decisions? How do you help her get through surgery? And how can you keep her encouraged?

- **Remind her you love her, not just her body (if appropriate).** If you are the spouse or significant other, her breast cancer may challenge the strength of your intimate relationship due to the range of physical changes her body will undergo. So, one of the best things you can do is remind her of all the ways you love her for who she is, not only the attributes of her physical appearance. Her body image is very fragile right now. If you can offer reassurance of your acceptance, that's one less anxiety-provoking issue that she'll have to contend with right now.

- **Let her make her own surgical decisions (with your unconditional support).** If she is offered a choice of surgical procedures—a lumpectomy versus mastectomy—don't impose your personal preference on her or attempt to persuade her because you think she may be particularly vulnerable or indecisive right now. Don't attempt to take over. And if she does ask you, be flexible. If you pressure her one way or the other, you may be asking for problems down the road—either guilt if she doesn't follow your suggestion and you end up with intimacy issues, or resentment and anger if she does and later suffers a recurrence but might have taken a different path the first time. All you should do is listen patiently, be a sounding board to help her arrive at her own decision, and provide unconditional support once she's decided. It is her body and she has to live with it for the rest of her life.

- **Be the hospital traffic cop for well-wishers.** If she has a lumpectomy, your job is fairly simple here. Since she may be in the hospital for only a day, one of you in her inner circle—her spouse, a family member, a friend—should plan to be there for the duration. Be in her room when she arrives from recovery, and leave when she goes to sleep. Be at her beck and call. Then be there the next day until she's discharged, and you can help her get home. The only "trafficking" you may have to do is monitoring telephone calls from well-wishers. Even if she's awake and not trying to sleep, she might not feel like reliving the experience for everyone who calls to ask, "So, how did it go?" If she's had a mastectomy, your job will be more extensive, as you'll have to help schedule visitors according to her energy level and emotional state.

- **Avoid the hero worship syndrome.** Once she is out of the hospital and on her way to recovery, don't put her on a pedestal. Avoid the temptation to tell her how brave she is to be going through all this. She's not a hero. She didn't have a choice. She's just getting through it, one day at a time. She'll be much more comforted if you tell her how bad you feel that she's having to go through this, and if she ever needs a shoulder to cry on, yours is ready and waiting.

- **Hone your financial management skills.** Help her through the financial and insurance quagmire she may have to contend with, beginning with surgery and through to the completion of treatment. It can be daunting. Offer to set up a record-keeping system that will be simple to follow and track payments made. Call the insurance companies to get confirmation of required procedures or challenge coverage levels if they are not satisfactory. Track the invoices and bills paid on a monthly basis. This is one project you can take off her plate.

- **Learn to interpret pathology reports.** If she is too overwhelmed, intimidated, or scared to read and interpret her own pathology report, help her along. It is a terrifying experience, a harsh dose of reality, to stare at a piece of paper on which the words "malignant cells" are associated with your name. However, in order to understand what her health care team is recommending in terms of follow-up treatments and why, she needs to know what the pathology report says.

Educate yourself enough so that you can accompany her to her doctor's visit when the pathology report will be discussed and be prepared to ask appropriate questions.

- **Provide uplifting reading (and viewing) material.** As with anyone who is sick or laid up temporarily, good books or videos are a welcome distraction and fill those often long voids of time. However, for the breast cancer patient, you need to do a little editing. Make sure that whatever you bring her is uplifting, inspirational, and joyful. The last thing she needs now is an angst-ridden story about a lost loved one. Funny movies are perfect as laughter encourages healing. Only happy endings need apply.

- **Encourage milestones.** While she will probably have several milestone events in her own mind that signal her progress on the road to recovery, help her along. Perhaps she already knows it's her return to work or a special family outing or celebration that she wants to look good at. Add something else special to her agenda. Schedule an activity or event that you can do together that will make her feel like she's back to her old self.

PART III
TREATMENT

CHAPTER 6

Deciphering Treatment Alternatives

A rmed with the facts from your pathology report and informa-tion gleaned from consultations with your health care team, you will shortly enter the treatment phase of this cancer journey. However, you may be a bit mystified about the seeming plethora of choices out there and why certain doctors are making specific rec-ommendations. This section will arm you with a bit of information to help you decipher all the alternatives you may have been bom-barded with:

- A discussion of *Chemotherapy and Radiation* and the theory behind each protocol, and
- Overviews of *Tamoxifen* and *Arimidex*, and how these hormone treatments can eliminate any cancer cells from your body.

CHEMOTHERAPY AND RADIATION: THE THEORY BEHIND EACH

What's the Difference? Chemotherapy Is Systemic, Radiation the Local Cleanup.

In your postsurgery discussions about what treatments you should undergo to ensure that the cancer is gone from your body, you will be faced with decisions about chemotherapy, radiation, or both. So what's the difference?

Chemotherapy is the therapeutic use of a variety of chemicals—given intravenously or orally—to systemically destroy any cancerous-type cells that might be lingering anywhere in your body. "Systemic" means chemo travels through your bloodstream to most cells in your body. If any cancerous cells have passed through your underarm lymph nodes and traveled to other parts of your body, those cells might lie dormant forever, or grow into tumors elsewhere in your body. The three most common places that breast cancer cells tend to anchor and rear their ugly heads at a later date are the lungs, liver, and bones, but they can also travel to other lymph nodes and even to the brain.

If you were lymph-node negative, you may wonder why oncologists still might recommend chemotherapy. I certainly did. "Why do I need that? They removed the cancer by surgery and it's all gone!" Well, yes, hopefully in fact, in the majority of women, that is the truth. But for a few, they just don't know. In addition to the lymph system, a second way that cancerous cells can travel to other parts of the body is through the bloodstream. However, there is no blood test available today that can definitively indicate if microscopic cancerous cells have been carried elsewhere, so there's no way to pinpoint exactly which women fall into that minority. Therefore, oncologists might recommend chemo for you as an aggressive, proactive move in their concern about your long-term health. This preventative approach to chemotherapy is called "adjuvant" therapy.

Radiation, as opposed to the systemic nature of chemotherapy, is a localized treatment—to the chest area only—used following a lumpectomy. (If you underwent a mastectomy, your doctor may or may not recommend radiation to the chest wall.) Essentially, radiation therapy is high-intensity X rays directed in many small dosages to the entire breast area, as a means to destroy any remaining cancerous cells left in the breast following surgery. So now you're wondering why you need radiation if your surgery resulted in "clear" margins? Again, like chemo, it's just another form of insurance. Theoretically, with clear margins, all the cancer was removed through surgery. However, with a lumpectomy, part of the breast organ remains in your body, and no doctor can tell you whether that organ contains any remaining stray cells not part of the original tumor or malformed cells that might become cancer, just the way your original cancer grew. Radiation hopefully destroys any suspicious cells that might remain.

Chemotherapy: A PacMan Game Going On inside Your Body.

So now we know that the theory behind chemotherapy is systemic—that it destroys any lingering cancer cells in your body. So, now how does it work? Think of the chemo "agent" as those little creatures in that PacMan game that gobble up anything in their path and sweep them away. Chemotherapy agents are chemicals that interfere with the replication of rapidly dividing cells at different stages of cell growth. Administering a series of treatments of the same or a different drug over time ensures the chemo gets all cancer cells as they enter different phases of their growth cycle.

So, the chemo PacMan is programmed to look for fast-growing cells in your body. That's fine, except there's one slight problem here. The chemo PacMan is rather indiscriminate, and not only does he gobble up any remaining cancer cells, but he snatches other fast-growing cells in your body: hair follicles, gastrointestinal lining, blood-forming cells, skin cells, and ovaries. Note that the destruction, or "toxicity," to these cells accounts for the most common side effects of chemotherapy that you hear and read about:

- *Hair*—possible thinning or loss, not only on your head, but all over your body.
- *Gastrointestinal lining*—appetite changes, nausea, irregular digestion, mouth sores, dry throat, etc.
- *Red and white blood cells and platelets* (all produced by the bone marrow)—greater susceptibility to infection and disease, hence the terms *immunosuppressed* and *immune-compromised,* as well as anemia and bleeding tendencies.
- *Skin*—dryness, sun sensitivity, pigment changes.
- *Ovaries*—menopausal-like symptoms, either temporary or permanent.

So, what's the good news? The first four fast-growing cells regenerate themselves fairly quickly and come back to normal. The hair and gastrointestinal cells return to normal once you're finished with treatment. Your blood cells need to regenerate each treatment cycle, so you won't be given your next treatment until your blood counts are back to normal. (You can't risk destroying your entire immune system!) Any skin pigment changes, such as freckling or sun sensitivity, should fade over time and dryness is temporary. However, your ovaries, depending on your age and how close you are to natural menopause, may or may not return to normal (more on this later).

There are also other toxicities not related to interference with rapidly growing cells, but instead are specific to individual drugs. (See "A Note from the Oncologist: Most Common Side Effects of Most Common Drugs.")

A NOTE FROM THE ONCOLOGIST

R̶x̶ *Most Common Side Effects of Most Common Drugs*

The most important thing to remember here is to stay positive! Unpleasant side effects may occur, but any given side effect is unlikely. In fact, an entire new "generation" of drugs is available today that is given in conjunction with chemotherapy to counteract the potential negative side effects. Among others, these range from antinausea drugs to injections that stimulate white blood cell growth so the time period that you are at risk of infection during your treatment cycle is shortened. Undergoing chemotherapy today is much more tolerable than the stories you heard about even ten years ago. So, don't scare yourself into expecting that just because you will be given some of the drugs on this list, that you will suffer from all the effects. Every body reacts differently, and your experience will be unique, so take it one day at a time. The list below (and for that matter, the entire section of managing the physical side effects of treatment) is just to keep you aware of what might happen, and what you can do to alleviate it. We want you to approach this phase of treatment with your eyes wide open—with a realistic, but not alarmist, perspective. So the most common drugs and their effects are the following.

- ***Adriamycin (doxorubicin).*** More common side effects are hair loss, nausea, mouth sores, and low blood counts. Less common but more worrisome is a problem with the regulation of a specific heart valve. While the risk is dosage dependent, for the standard treatment regimen, it is actually less than 1 percent. Anyone receiving this drug will go for cardiac testing and be monitored appropriately for the duration.
- ***Cytoxan (cyclophosphamide).*** More common effects include metallic mouth taste while the drug is being administered, and later nausea, appetite changes, hair loss, and low blood counts. Also irregularities in your menstrual cycle can occur, and as total dosages increase, fertility declines, while the likelihood of premature menopause increases. Rarely, there can be toxicity to the bladder (to prevent this, drink plenty of fluids) and metabolic abnormalities.
- ***Ellence (epirubicin).*** Long used in Europe in place of Adriamycin, this drug may have less cardiac toxicity. Some oncologists may prefer it to Adriamycin. It is similar in its toxicities.
- ***Methotrexate.*** Generally without toxicity other than nausea, mouth sores, and low blood counts. In rare cases, the liver can be injured.
- ***5-Fluorouracil.*** Also fairly well tolerated. More common effects are mouth sores, nausea, appetite changes, and diarrhea. Rarely, skin darkening or pigment changes can occur.
- ***Taxol (paclitaxel).*** The primary concern is about an allergic reaction, so everyone receiving this drug gets pretreatment with antihistamines and anti-inflammatory drugs. Common effects are hair loss, nausea, low blood counts, and less frequently, neurological side effects, such as weakness, numbness, and tingling (which may be

temporary during treatment or more permanent, depending on dosages and duration).

- **Taxotere (docetaxel).** Similar allergic reactions to Taxol may occur. Swelling in the legs and fluid buildup, sometimes in the lungs, can be a problem. Nail changes and tear duct problems may also occur.
- **Herceptin (trastuzumab).** This is a monoclonal antibody against HER2-neu. There may be allergic reactions. Additionally, there can be cardiac damage (generally reversible), so follow-up with a cardiologist will be arranged. Because of this potential, it is never given together with doxorubicin (see above).

Other more general side effects of chemotherapy may include temporary memory loss, fatigue, and depression, induced by a complex interaction of chemical, physical, and emotional factors.

Radiation: Imagine an Electronic Weed Killer in Carefully Measured Dosages.

So if chemotherapy is systemic and radiation is localized, then how exactly does radiation work? And how do the doctors determine what to radiate? Consider cancer as a weed growing in your breast. While surgery may remove the visible part of the weed, including what you think is the root, there still may be seedlings scattered around the remaining tissue. Even if you had clear margins, there may still be some "stray" cancer cells left behind that were outside the margin. So, radiation is intended to eliminate any stray cells left behind.

Radiation works by attacking the key characteristic that distinguishes cancer from healthy cells. Essentially, radiation is an extremely high-intensity X ray that cuts through a cell and damages its DNA structure, that genetic coding that instructs a cell to replicate, particularly while rapidly dividing (as cancer cells do). While healthy cells have the ability to repair themselves, cancer cells only have the capacities to replicate, attack, or destruct. So, incapable of repair, the cancer cell dies. Over the years, radiation oncologists have determined the optimal dosage of radiation that kills cancer but allows healthy tissue to repair itself to normal over time.

A major breast study by the National Surgical Adjuvant Breast and Bowel Project (NSABP) indicated that the rate of local recurrence in women who underwent lumpectomies may be 35–40 percent without radiation, but drops dramatically to 7–12 percent with radiation. That is why today radiation is considered standard, mandatory treatment following lumpectomy. You don't have a choice. If you had a lumpectomy, then generally radiation is part of the package. If you had a mastectomy, your doctor may suggest radiation as part of treatment, with a focus on the remaining breast skin and chest wall area.

Depending on a variety of factors, your radiation oncologist will determine what areas radiation should cover. Taking into account your physical anatomy (e.g., the structure of your breast area), the size of your tumor, and extent of lymph node involvement, if any, your doctor may recommend radiating areas that extend beyond the remaining breast tissue, such as the chest wall, the axillary lymph node area (in your underarm), or even the supraclavicular nodes (in the neck area).

First Comes Chemo . . . Then a Sandwich?

If it is recommended that you undergo both chemotherapy and radiation, you will hear many different opinions and much confusing information about which order they should be given and when. Some doctors believe that certain chemotherapy agents can exacerbate any tissue damage from radiation, so they avoid concurrent treatments. So which comes first? While many doctors today recommend chemo first to eliminate any stray cancer cells systemically, and then radiation as localized follow-up, you will hear different versions of this. One is even called a sandwich, where the six or so weeks of radiation are "sandwiched" in the middle of the chemo regimen. So, what's best for you? You need to balance the opinions of your doctors with what works best for your schedule, access to treatment facilities, and physical stamina (how much your body can handle).

Cocktails? Aren't Those for Celebrations?

Any chemotherapy recommended for you will most likely be a "cocktail" or a mixture of two to four different drugs. Why? Because each drug acts in a different way to get at cancer cells. Some attack the speed at which the cell replicates, some increase the rate of cell mortality, and some affect how cells stick together, which keeps them from straying from the original tumor site. Said differently, chemotherapy either kills the cell directly or corrupts the cell's ability to divide and replicate. Furthermore, some cancer cells may be resistant to one drug but not another. And last, using drugs in combination also lets drugs work sequentially on the same cell, so it is attacked on all fronts simultaneously, and one drug may actually enhance the effectiveness of another.

A Port: A Device to Deliver Chemotherapy Drugs, Not a Shelter for a Boat in a Storm.

I've always thought of a port as someplace that a ship can pull into to avoid the ravages of a storm. In chemo jargon, it's the heart of the storm. For a variety of reasons, your oncologist might suggest that you receive drugs through a "vascular access device," commonly called a "port." It's a small device that gets surgically implanted (through outpatient day surgery) under your skin on your chest. If you will be receiving chemotherapy in many doses, if the specific drugs are known to be "tough" on your veins, or if your veins appear difficult to access, your oncologist might recommend a port. Decide carefully, as there are benefits and drawbacks. The greatest benefit is the ease of administering drugs, for both the nurses and for you not to have your arm pricked in so many different places. However, the greatest drawback, in addition to more surgery, is the tendency for the port site to get infected or clot, and therefore, have to be removed in the midst of treatment. And given your immuno-suppressed state, you don't need an extra infection right now. If your doctor suggests a port, determine if the benefits outweigh the drawbacks for you.

TAMOXIFEN: THE ORIGINAL HORMONE OPTION

And Then There's the Tamoxifen Factor . . . Locking Up Your Health.

If your pathology report indicated that you had "estrogen-receptor positive" (ER+) cell types, then you may be a candidate for tamoxifen in addition to or instead of chemotherapy. Since estrogen-positive cells means that your cancer cells are fueled by estrogen, then theoretically if estrogen can be prevented from attaching to any remaining traces of breast cancer cells, the risk of your cancer returning is reduced. Tamoxifen acts on breast cancer cells as an "anti-estrogen." ER+ cancer cells need to "lock" on to estrogen in order to grow and thrive (the estrogen acts as the "key" to turn on the cell to flourish). But if tamoxifen is introduced into your body, any bad cells will "lock" onto the tamoxifen instead of estrogen, so they simply die and get washed out of your body, rather than growing into tumors.

Tamoxifen is taken in pill form daily for several years following your surgery. If your doctor proposes it, it's worth serious consideration. It's also an inspiration to illustrate how quickly new treatments are being developed for this disease. Only ten short years ago, tamoxifen was considered experimental. Today it's standard therapy.

Side Effects and Risks of Tamoxifen . . . but the Clinical Trade-Off Is Unparalleled Today.

Tamoxifen is an important treatment for patients with ER+ cancer cells, particularly postmenopausal, but for many pre-menopausal women as well. Presently, there is no drug that can match the clinical experience of tamoxifen in the treatment (and even prevention) of breast cancer. (See "A Note from the Doctor: Tamoxifen Treatment versus Prevention: Getting Past the Media Hype"). As you will see below, however, a new drug, Arimidex, is a viable new alternative. So if your doctor recommends it, and you confirm its importance in your care independently, then take it without trepidation (remember, it's now considered safe enough to use preventively *without* cancer). Just be aware that while it really is very benign compared to chemotherapy, there are still potential rare side effects. Mild nausea might occur at the beginning, and hot flashes and other menopausal symptoms are possible. The more serious potential side effects—a slight propensity to develop blood clots, cataracts, even uterine cancer—can all be monitored and screened for by your doctors over the longer term. No doubt you experienced a moment of panic as you noticed uterine cancer on this list. Does this mean you'd be trading one cancer for another? No! The survival benefits of tamoxifen outweigh the very slight risk of uterine cancer by 20 to 1.

To Wait or Not to Wait.

When to begin tamoxifen in the course of your treatment process is open to debate, and different doctors will have different preferences. Some women will begin immediately after chemotherapy and/or radiation are completed, while others wait to give their bodies a reprieve from the toxic effects of treatments. If they let their body return to normal, cleansed of the effects of chemotherapy before starting tamoxifen, they can then more clearly determine if and when any side effects might be due to tamoxifen.

And If You Do, Don't Forget the Birth Control.

If you do decide to go on tamoxifen, and you are sexually active and not yet past permanent menopause, you must use some type of birth control. Although you may experience menopausal-like symptoms because tamoxifen acts like an antiestrogen, you may still be capable of getting pregnant, and it is contraindicated to get pregnant while on tamoxifen. However, once you finish tamoxifen, any drug-related, menopausal-like symptoms should dissipate and you should be clear to become pregnant should you decide to do so (given that your oncologist is comfortable with your decision based on your health history and the entire set of risk factors).

Add a Bone Density Scan to Your Medical Portfolio.

As you probably know, as women age, particularly after menopause, they are at increasing risk of osteoporosis, or thinning of the bones, which can result in debilitating fractures. And since tamoxifen acts as an antiestrogen in your body, it may have the same effect as the hormonal changes associated with menopause. However, the jury is still divided on the potential effect of tamoxifen on your bones. Early indications showed that perhaps tamoxifen has beneficial effects on bone density. However, more recently, there's been noise about loss of bone density. Ask your doctor whether you should have a baseline bone density scan against which later measurements can be taken to determine if tamoxifen is accelerating bone loss in your body.

A Note from the Doctor

℞ *Tamoxifen Treatment versus Prevention: Getting Past the Media Hype*

The clinical finding that tamoxifen not only reduced recurrences of breast cancer when given as an adjuvant treatment, but also reduced the incidence of new cancers in the opposite, or "contralateral," breast, has led some of the country's leading researchers to study the role of tamoxifen in the *prevention* of breast cancer in women at high risk.

In the monumental Breast Cancer Prevention Trial, a project funded by the NCI's National Surgical Adjuvant Breast and Bowel Project (NSABP), more than 13,000 women who were at risk for breast cancer were given either tamoxifen or a placebo on a randomized basis. The factors determining relative risk were: number of first-degree relatives (mother, sister, daughter) affected by breast cancer, the number of previous benign breast biopsies, age when delivered first live birth, and the presence of any atypical growth of cells.

In May 1998, the study code was "broken" to reveal overwhelming success. Tamoxifen reduced the incidence of breast cancer by approximately 50 percent, the first time that any medication could actually be demonstrated to reduce the risk of cancer! Needless to say, such success has caused significant media flurry, where it's been touted as the wonder drug that cures cancer and cancer-to-be in all women. Take a step back, and don't get caught in the hype. Only by evaluating the specifics of your situation with your doctor can you determine if it's right for you—either as an adjuvant treatment or as a preventative. Many further studies have confirmed the efficacy of tamoxifen in preventing breast cancer 1 for women at risk.

AROMATASE INHIBITORS: THE OTHER HORMONAL OPTION

Aromatase inhibitors are antiestrogen drugs with a completely different method of action and side effect profile than tamoxifen. There are three drugs presently in this class: Arimidex (anastrozole), Femara (letrozole), and Aromasin (exemestane). A trial called the ATAC trial (an acronym for Arimidex, Tamoxifen, Alone or in Combination) demonstrated that for postmenopausal patients with estrogen receptor positive tumors, there was an advantage for using Arimidex alone versus using tamoxifen or the combination. Similarly, a trial called the BIG 1-98 trial demonstrated an advantage of Femara over tamoxifen in postmenopausal patients. As such, Arimidex and Femara have become standard for these patients after chemotherapy (and radiation therapy, if given). Your doctor will choose which one. There is also data for the use of Aromasin for patients who become menopausal during treatment, with a split of tamoxifen for two to three years, followed by Aromasin, to total five years. Finally, for patients who become menopausal toward the end of their use of tamoxifen, there is data to suggest that an additional five years of an aromatase inhibitor is helpful in preventing recurrence.

Aromatase inhibitors act by cutting off the enzyme (you guessed it, it is called "aromatase") that allows the adrenal glands, fat cells, and other organs in the body that still make estrogen from doing so, thus eliminating the last tiny bit of estrogen in the body (the ovaries are already "off," remember). This is different from tamoxifen, which has some pro-estrogen-like qualities (like being good for bones).

Aromatase inhibitors are well tolerated, with fewer of the hot flashes, none of the potential toxicity to the uterus, and less propensity to cause clotting. They are not protective of bones, however, so the risk of osteoporosis and osteopenia (less calcium in the bones) is greater. Your doctor will therefore want to follow your bone density studies. He or she will likely place you on calcium and vitamin D, and may need to consider other drugs to strengthen bones, if necessary.

Despite the mild drawbacks of the aromatase inhibitors, they have improved the care of postmenopausal women, and represent a substantial step forward in the armamentarium against breast cancer. Your doctor will help decide which aromatase inhibitor is best for you.

CHAPTER 7

Managing Treatments: Chemotherapy and Radiation

Okay, so you're suffering from research overload, have decided upon a treatment regimen, and are ready to take the plunge. This chapter will cover three aspects of how to manage treatments, including:

- The *Process* of getting through the daily grind of chemotherapy and/or radiation treatment, day in and day out.
- All the potential *Physical Side Effects* and changes that your body might undergo with chemotherapy or radiation, with head-to-toe advice on how to minimize your discomfort and maximize your wellness.
- Your *Work* schedule, and how to create whatever arrangement works best for you at this time.

MANAGING THE PROCESS OF CHEMOTHERAPY TREATMENTS

If you were like the majority of women with early-stage breast cancer, you were rolling along in life feeling great until some doctor told you that you were sick with cancer. And just to make sure you never get sick again, they pump you full of drugs that make you feel horrible. Makes a lot of sense, right? Sorry, but unfortunately that's the way it often works. This chapter will help you endure, and perhaps even find some humor in managing, both the treatment routine and the physical changes that may occur as the chemotherapy demolishes those fastest-growing cells in your body (refer back to Chapter 6 for a discussion of the theory behind chemotherapy). Remember, all except any stray cancer cells repair themselves.

Four Sessions, Six, or More? The Science behind the Number of Sessions.

Research studies over many years have determined the optimal way to administer chemotherapy drugs to provide the maximum dosage that can be tolerated by the body (without permanent damage to healthy tissues) and, therefore, the greatest chance of killing any remaining cancer cells. Depending on what combination of drugs your oncologist recommends, you may have four, six, or eight treatment sessions spaced approximately three to four weeks apart, or weekly for two weeks, then off for two weeks. The time periods between these treatment days allow your body to recover from any damage to healthy cells, such as white blood cells in the bone marrow. The drugs will be administered to you either by intravenous drip, which can take anywhere from thirty minutes to a few hours, or orally in pill form. Chemotherapy can be administered on an outpatient basis at a hospital, in a special treatment clinic, or even in your doctor's office.

Monthly Calendars Will Become Irrelevant. Manage Your Life in "Chemo Cycle" Increments.

Depending on your doctors, the treatment protocol, and your body's reaction to the specific type of chemotherapy you'll receive, you will be put on a treatment schedule, as discussed above. Forget about planning your life on any "normal" time period like weeks or months right now. Rearrange it according to your chemo cycle. After a cycle or two, you will know that you have days that you feel fine, and days that you're not so fine, days that you are more energetic or much weaker than usual, days with a hearty appetite and days you don't even want to smell food, even days that your white blood cell counts are low, so you are more susceptible to infections.

(More on this later, but your doctors may track your blood counts by drawing blood periodically through your treatment cycle.) Make your plans accordingly. Don't plan a full day of work followed by a dinner party on a day you know it may be difficult to even drag yourself out of bed. Don't go to the movie theater, shopping mall, or other indoor places with crowds of people on days that your blood counts might be low.

A Preface to Treatment Day: Drink, Drink, Drink (Sorry, Not Alcohol)!

If you've never been a water drinker before, now is the time to become one. One of the best ways to get the chemotherapy flushing through your body and out as soon as it's done its job is to drink a lot of water—more than you ever thought you were capable of. If you feel you've drunk enough to irrigate a desert, then you're finally drinking enough. Drink at least eight to ten glasses of water per day:

- Two to three days before treatment—to get your kidneys moving and prepared to flush the drugs through your body (some drugs can cause kidney damage if they do not flush through properly).
- Three to four days after treatment—to flush the drugs through; to prevent possible dehydration from any nausea; to minimize any digestive problems or constipation from the antinausea drugs or steroids.
- All the days in between—since your chemotherapy mixture is chemicals, it is very drying to the body in general. Drinking water will help prevent dry skin; dry, irritated eyes; dry throat; vaginal dryness; and dry anything else that you can imagine.

Treatment Day: Transform It into an Outing in Five Easy Steps.

Step 1. Bring Someone.

Instead of thinking, "Oh no, I have to go to the hospital for chemo today," make your chemotherapy day into a special outing of otherwise pleasant events. Bring a close friend, your spouse, or another relative with you. It passes the time in the waiting room before you see your oncologist, who generally checks to see how you tolerated the last session and whether you are physically okay to receive your next session of chemotherapy that day (e.g., sufficient blood count levels, no colds or infections). It also distracts you from getting worried and nervous about what might happen to your body this time, and it's a great chance to catch up on both old and new friendships. You'll have that rare time to talk without the everyday interruptions of kids, work, schedules, etc. And your friend or relative gets to see a bit of your life and understand what you are experiencing. In turn, it's amazing what they will reveal to you about their own lives, as they witness your current drama.

About two hours before you go in for treatment, eat a meal. Any nausea that you might experience from chemo will be minimized if you receive treatment on a full stomach. Make sure your meal includes breads and proteins. Stay away from fats, grease, and sugar.

Worried about finding someone willing to accompany you to treatment? Don't be. You probably won't even have to ask. I had more people volunteering to come with me than I had number of treatments—a very nice position to be in. It really makes you appreciate all those people who make your life so special.

Step 2. Bring a Few Things.

Just as you plan what to pack for a vacation, a little planning for your treatment visit makes the experience more tolerable. A few things to consider:

- Wear comfortable clothes as you want to be so relaxed that you can doze off if your treatment lasts a few hours. Make sure your sleeves can be rolled up easily for an IV needle.
- Bring a sweater, or a blanket, even if it's warm outside. Treatment areas, like hospitals, are often very cool to minimize bacteria and germs.
- Bring materials to pass the time and distract your mind. These might include lighthearted books, magazines, relaxation tapes or music with a Walkman, even a crossword puzzle—nothing too heavy or intense because you might not be able to concentrate all that well.

- Bring a snack. Since you might have to wait a long time to see your doctor and be treated, bring something to snack on to make sure your stomach is full when you start. Crackers, breads, or pretzels work best.
- Bring a notebook (or your "logbook") and a calendar. Use the notebook for any questions you need to ask your doctor. Use the calendar to record timing and dosages of any follow-up medications you might need to take for a few days afterward.
- Bring Popsicles or Fudgsicles! If you are being given Adriamycin, bring along something cold to suck on during its administration to lessen the chance of getting mouth sores. This tidbit of advice was actually the inspiration for this book!

Step 3. Leave Some Things Home (if You Ever Want to Use Them Again).

Chemotherapy treatment is a testament to the mind's power of association. You will forever associate certain things with this experience. To this day, whenever I visit the doctor for a checkup, just passing the sign to the treatment area makes me nauseous and lightheaded. I still can't fathom eating another Popsicle or Fudgsicle ever again in my life. Some women say that if they've chewed on ice, it takes a long time to be able to put ice in their drinks again. And some go so far as developing an aversion to the color red if they received Adriamycin, since the drug is dark red in color. If there is anything that you want to use ever again—be it your favorite music tape or book—think about leaving it home. Bring things you can dispose of when you're through.

Step 4. Distract Yourself in the Treatment Waiting Area.

On your first visit to a chemotherapy treatment center, you might panic and begin to think of yourself as a "cancer patient." You'll get frightened at all the frail-looking, balding women with scarves or wigs, and wonder why you are there with all these sick people. Don't despair. Keep your chin up by telling yourself that everyone has a different situation, that being a "cancer patient" is not your permanent identity and that you'll be fine. Distract yourself. Try to determine whose hair is real, and whose is a wig. You'll see how difficult it is to tell the difference, which means that yours probably looks pretty good! If you don't have do endure the hair loss trauma, find another type of guessing game to distract yourself. Take the time to notice any artwork on the wall. How often do you do that?

Step 5. Go Home, but Make a Few Stops?

Regardless of whether someone accompanies you to treatment, as suggested in Step 1, definitely make sure that someone is "on call" to pick you up and take you home. There are two good reasons for this. First, your physical reaction to treatment will vary each and every time, so just because you feel great once doesn't mean you will always feel great. You might be weak, headachy, or sleepy, and not want to drive yourself or even deal with public transportation. Second, from the standpoint of making this day into an outing, you need someone to celebrate the fact that you're done with one more treatment. If you feel okay, go out for lunch, dinner, or simply a cup of coffee to a place that you enjoy. Perhaps even make an appointment for a manicure, facial, massage, or anything else that makes you feel good. Treat yourself. You deserve it. If you don't feel so great, plan what you'll do in a couple of days to treat yourself.

Nurses Are a True Source of Comfort.

You'll be spending a great deal of time with oncology nurses during your chemotherapy treatments, and you'll find them to be a great source of knowledge, and comfort as well. You might ask to meet with them even before you settle on an oncologist and start treatment, so that you can judge whether: (a) they will provide you with tricks of the trade for mitigating side effects (like sucking on Popsicles and all the other advice in this book), (b) they have the time and patience to attend to your needs and questions, and (c) you find them compassionate and comforting enough to trust them to stick a needle in your vein. They often become your friends.

Chemo Today or Not? Only Your Blood Counts Know for Sure.

After your first treatment, all subsequent treatments will begin with drawing blood to determine if your white blood cell count has rebounded to a "normal" level and your immune system is strong enough for the next dose. In other words, if your prior treatment destroyed too many blood cells, and your body has not repaired itself sufficiently, your doctor will most likely postpone your treatment for a few days to give your body additional time to regenerate those cells. Otherwise, you risk running down your immune system too far and being too susceptible to infection that you wouldn't be able to fight. This can be disappointing in a bizarre way, since you've emotionally prepared yourself for the treatment and were looking forward to getting one more over with. However, considering the alternative—a potentially life-threatening infection—be glad that your doctors are monitoring you so carefully.

Keep a Calendar. It Becomes Easier to Forecast the Future.

As soon as you go home, use your calendar to record any physical side effects you experience from this treatment session. (This might be part of your health care team log book; see page 64.) Include questions to ask your doctor on your next visit (if not urgent). Keeping track of what happens to you during the first twelve hours, twenty-four hours, three days after treatment, throughout your entire cycle, will help your doctors determine if something is becoming serious, or if there are adjustments they can make to your medication to prevent such side effects from occurring again. For example, if you felt okay for two days, and then had some nausea on Day 3, they might keep you on antinausea medication for a day or two longer. Alternatively, if you got constipated after three or four days but not particularly nauseous, they might switch you to a milder medication that is easier on your digestive system. Being able to predict what might happen to you will also relieve some of your anxiety, and aid you in mentally pushing through it. If you know that you are likely to be pretty miserable on Day 3, you can be prepared for it and be comforted that it will last only twenty-four hours, and then you'll feel better.

Your Oncologist (and Radiation Oncologist) Will Become Your Travel Agent.

I don't easily sit still, either in my professional or in my personal life. But I was forced to sit still, or at least sit in one city, for the duration of treatment. During chemotherapy, your doctor will probably not let you travel far from his or her sight. If you develop a fever, or some other unexpected side effect, he will want you within an hour or so of the hospital. Side effects, for the most part, will go away on their own. But in rare situations, they can get serious and when they do, they do so quickly. In addition, you can't show up at just any hospital and assume they'll know how to treat you because they will not have your medical history and files. Be sure to discuss any travel plans with your doctor. If you are allowed to travel, you might want to identify a nearby hospital that could treat you if necessary, and have any important records faxed to an oncologist who would be prepared to care for you.

I can attest to the seriousness of unexpected side effects. I actually had an allergic reaction to one of the drugs in my chemotherapy regimen which landed me in the emergency room within two hours of initial symptoms, and luckily I was close to home. My doctor later informed me that it could have been life-threatening.

Be Prepared for "Little Scares."

Inevitably, you will experience "little scares" that loom very large at the moment, but you will get past them, and in the scheme of life they will become rather insignificant. Since each and every person responds differently to all aspects of treatment—radiation. chemotherapy, drugs to mitigate side effects—no doctor can tell you exactly what will happen to *you* personally. Therefore, you'll just have to handle these "little scares" as your body decides to define them for you.

One of my little scares seemed life-threatening to me at the time. One day shortly after my first chemotherapy, I was walking down the street—probably too fast and in weather too warm to be outside—and my vision started to blank out. I got light-headed, started seeing white spots, and immediately panicked, thinking, "Oh my God, they never told me that chemo can make you blind! Or worse, maybe I'm having a stroke!" Well, to make a long story short, after a quick but scary trip to the emergency room, I was basically fine.

Simply put, the chemotherapy had affected the blood cells that carried oxygen to my body, and I wasn't getting enough oxygen circulating to keep up the energetic pace I was moving at that day. So did I get similar symptoms thereafter? Sure, but the next time I knew what was happening to me. And when my treatment finished, they went away, just as the doctors promised.

Put Someone (or Two or Three or Four People) in Charge of Your Social Calendar.

One of the best pieces of advice I heard on how to get through the very long months of chemotherapy was to select a social committee so you have activities and events to look forward to and brighten your day in the midst of the drudgery of treatment. Choose four of your most creative, spontaneous, fun friends, and inform them that they are in charge of making sure that once a week you have something to look forward to. It doesn't matter if they work as a group (if they are friendly with one another), or if they each take responsibility for one week of each month. And it doesn't really matter what you do. It can be as simple as coming over with dinner and a rental movie (as long as it's uplifting), a walk in a nearby park, or a manicure (if your blood counts permit). All that matters is that you can anticipate enjoyment and you don't have to expend any energy to plan it.

MANAGING PHYSICAL SIDE EFFECTS: HEAD-TO-TOE ADVICE

Since chemotherapy is a systemic treatment that theoretically travels to every cell in your body, there are many, many potential side effects, some very common, some extremely rare. The biggest unknown of all, though, is how your particular body will react. Some of you will breeze through treatment and wonder why I have dedicated so many pages to side effects, while others may have a tougher go of it. Regardless of your experience, hopefully you will all find something helpful in this section that provides head-to-toe advice, from ways to manage hair loss to mouth and skin care, to minimizing nausea and maintaining appetite, to controlling menopausal symptoms, among other things. And through it all, should you experience anything that is unusual or different about your body, do not hesitate to call your doctor.

A NOTE FROM ALL THE DOCTORS

R̶x **Eleven Reasons to Call the Doctor . . . and When to Leave Him or Her Alone**

While this section offers you a fairly comprehensive overview of what may happen to you, so you can anticipate it, handle it, and minimize any discomfort or anxiety, there are times when it is imperative to call the doctor immediately. By not doing so, you could risk serious infection, or damage to otherwise healthy organs and tissue. Pick up the phone immediately if or when:

- You have a fever, sweats, or chills—anything that signals your body temperature is off kilter (note that each doctor will give you a different "threshold" for what a fever might be—the most important thing is how you feel, and not your precise temperature).
- You have a skin rash that itches, burns, or swells—anywhere, including redness around your surgical site(s).
- You experience shortness of breath.
- You are so nauseous that you can't keep water down and are becoming dehydrated.
- You have other gastrointestinal problems such as loose bowels, stomach pain, or constipation.
- You develop gynecological discomfort such as burning/itching during urination or vaginal discharge.
- Your leg(s)—arm(s)—swell, or become tender.
- You have significant, sustained pain—anywhere.
- You have significant loss of appetite, listlessness, or fatigue associated with extreme sadness or depression.

- You are confused about how to take any medicine you were given (don't ever guess).
- You have a question about your care or condition that wasn't addressed at your last doctor's visit (either you just plain forgot to ask, or you didn't quite understand the doctor's explanation when you did ask).

However, when in doubt, if you are even thinking of calling, call! Every body is different, and will react to treatment in its own way. If you just feel lousy, or notice anything unusual or abnormal, don't hesitate to call. That's why doctors wear beepers! So you see, the category of "when to leave him or her *alone*" has *no* entries.

Coping with Hair Loss

Find a Wig Stylist and Make a "Prechemo" Visit. We're Lucky They're Back in Style.

Believe it or not, wigs are in style these days. And that's good news for those of us who will lose our hair from chemotherapy. Finding a good wig stylist is only a few questions away. A few places to ask: your hairdresser, any actor/actress friends, your medical oncologist, chemotherapy nurses, social workers at the hospital where you are being treated, other women you know who have been through this, or your support group (if you are involved with one). If all else fails, you can always call your local chapter of the American Cancer Society.

If it is nearly certain that you will lose your hair from your treatment (e.g., Adriamycin-based regimens), visit the wig fitter you've chosen before you begin chemotherapy, so they can find you a wig that most closely resembles your natural hairstyle (if that's what you want, and choose not to use this as an opportunity to change your hairstyle). Even if you are on a treatment regimen where you may only have gradual or partial hair loss (e.g., CMF), you might find comfort by visiting a wig fitter and having one picked out and ready to go, in the event that you need it.

Fear of Hair Loss? Just Get Buzzed.

At first, the thought of losing your hair can be terrifying, almost more so than chemotherapy itself. I met women who have said flatly that they wouldn't go through chemotherapy if they'd lose their hair. But remember the long-term goal—to get rid of any remaining cancer cells in the body. Plus, hair often comes back beautifully after chemo, often thick and wavy.

If you are receiving a drug that definitely causes total hair loss, shortly after your first treatment, your scalp may become very tender and uncomfortable. As soon as your hair starts coming out—and you'll definitely know it when you shower or as you brush it—give yourself a day or two to accept it. Then, visit your wig fitter to get your head shaved. Have your wig ready to go. Then just "get buzzed." It's much less traumatic and anxiety-provoking than the slow road to baldness. Yes, when my surgeon (a late-forties, balding man) told me to do this "if I had the guts," I thought he was out of his mind, and nearly had to run out of his office to the closest ladies room to pass out. But now, in retrospect, I think it takes more strength not to do it. Shaving your head lets you maintain control and dignity over how and when you lose your hair. And besides, your bathroom stays a lot cleaner!

But First, Empty the Vanity Cabinet.

Before you leave for your wig-fitting appointment, take a look in your bathroom vanity cabinet. Empty all hair products and hair accessories into a box that you'll put away until you have hair again. This might include hair dryers, rollers, curling irons, shampoos, styling gels, hairsprays, hair-coloring kits, brushes, combs, razors, wax, depilatories, etc. Not having to look at those items will make it easier to return home, and it's a good excuse to clean out your cabinet.

When It Comes to Wigs, 100% Natural Is Not Necessarily Better.

You might be advised by other women to cough up a fortune (which may not be covered by insurance) to purchase a natural hair wig. Not so fast. There are three general types of wigs on the market today, all with their own advantages and disadvantages. Determine which type works best for your lifestyle and pocketbook, based on the following advantages and drawbacks:

Wig Type	Advantages	Disadvantages
All-Natural Wigs	• Made from human hair, they are the most natural in terms of the basic look, the part, the feel, and how the hair moves. • Longest lasting since human hair doesn't dry out as quickly as synthetic. • Can be cut to your exact hairstyle. • Color can be matched most closely to your own. • Fit is most comfortable and coolest (may be important in hot weather).	• Requires almost daily styling by wig fitter or by you at home (with rollers and a cool blow dryer). • Not at all weather-resistant (you can still have "bad hair days"). • Costliest alternative.
Synthetic-Natural Blended Wigs	• Can be cut to your exact hairstyle. • Less costly than natural, with more natural features and feeling than all-synthetic. • Styling only required every 14–16 wearings. • Can still style yourself if desired (as opposed to synthetic, which cannot change styles). • Less sensitive to weather factors than all-natural (you'll only have a "bad hair day" if you get caught in the rain).	• Still requires maintenance by wig fitter. • Costlier than all-synthetic.

Wig Type	Advantages	Disadvantages
All-Synthetic Wigs	• Requires least maintenance, can be washed at home with baby shampoo about once a week, and will keep style • Indifference to weather conditions makes it appropriate for sports and outdoor activities (you'll never have a "bad hair days"). • Least costly option.	• Least flexibility to alter style or color to match your own. • Not as long-lasting as natural options, as hair dries out (about 3-month life span). • May be most artificial in color or appearance. • Not as comfortable as other options.

The Two-for-One Wig Special.

Depending on the type of chemotherapy you will receive, your doctor will provide you with a prescription for a hair prosthesis so the wig costs can be covered by your insurance company. But nobody will ever talk to you about *two* wigs. Yes, if you want to maintain your existing appearance, and not add scarves and hats to your wardrobe, you will need two wigs, not one. Why? Because depending on the type of hair in your wig, you will either need to wash it at home, or bring it into the salon to be washed and styled. In either case, you may want to wear one wig when the other is in "maintenance" mode.

You can get two identical wigs that replicate your hairstyle so you'll never be caught off-guard, or you can be creative. I opted for a formal "weekday" wig and a more casual "weekend" wig. My weekday wig was a natural-synthetic blend that replicated my exact haircut to maintain my appearance at work, while my "weekend" wig was an all-synthetic piece which let me do outdoor sports activities without worry. Who knows? It was so easy, I might decide at some point to revive the hassle-free "weekend" wig even with my "normal" hairstyle!

Wig or Hairpiece? When in Doubt, Go for the Wig.

This decision is not only physical, but emotional, so it's best to be prepared. If you are receiving a chemotherapy that will definitely cause complete hair loss, you will be given a prescription for a wig, which should be covered by insurance as a medical prosthesis. However, if you are undergoing treatment where you might experience gradual partial to complete hair loss (e.g., CMF), your doctor might recommend waiting to see if you lose hair, and get a hairpiece if it happens. A hairpiece is a smaller section of hair meant to supplement and blend in with your own hair. However, since the timing and extent of hair loss is so uncertain, your best option is still to just go get a wig. Consider it insurance for your emotional well-being. If, in fact, you do start to lose a lot of hair, you are prepared, both physically and emotionally.

A New Style? Only Your Hairdresser Knows for Sure.

If you want to keep your wig's style as close as possible to your prechemo hairstyle, then make sure you "capture" your existing style. Take pictures of your current hairstyle from the front, side, and back. Then bring them to your wig fitter and have them cut your wig to the exact style. However, while you might not want change right now, be open and flexible. Wig hair will not fall the same as natural hair across your head, or frame your face in precisely the same way. Trust your wig stylist to help you develop a similar, if not identical, style that flatters your face shape. Only your hairdresser will know the true you.

Maybe It's Time to Get Rid of That Kindergarten Pageboy.

If you're like me, you've been fairly, to say the least, unadventurous with your hair to date. I had maintained essentially the same basic pageboy that I sported in my kindergarten class picture. I knew it, it was safe, and it looked okay. Sure, it became more stylish than that first mug shot, and at times it's been slightly shorter, longer, or layered. And of course, I did go through my phase of perms. But I never tried anything radically different. Well, from here on out, after wearing wigs and hats for nearly a year, I'll be much more adventurous, stylish, and chic with my hair. I no longer fear not liking a hairstyle anymore. It always grows back. At least it's *my* hair.

Make Me a Redhead, Really?

Unless you opt for an all-natural wig, chances are that you'll have to alter your hair color somewhat, that you'll never find an exact match to your existing color. I am a dark brunette who always wished for more red highlights—the kind I used to get as a child, when I spent the entire summer outdoors in the sun. Well, I'm not wishing anymore. My weekend wig was full of fun red highlights so when my hair returned, I relied on my hairdresser to help keep my new reddish look!

Be adventurous. Use this time to experiment with color as well as style. You may have heard that your hair might come back a different texture from your original hair for the first year or so. Well, it might also come back a slightly different color. You may as well be prepared.

Silk Is for Slips and Underwear, Not Your Head.

If you decide to alternate between wigs and scarves, or forgo wigs altogether in favor of scarves and hats, don't rush out and treat yourself to a pretty new silk scarf (as I almost did). As much as you might feel like pampering yourself and treating yourself to silk scarves so you don't feel ugly, don't. They'll just slip right off your head. The secret? If you insist on wearing silk, wrap it over a cotton turban to hold it in place. Other options? Try cotton chamois, or even wool challis, and save the silk for your underwear.

Your Head Still Thinks You Have Hair. Shampoo It.

Believe it or not, if you lose your hair from drugs like Adriamycin or Taxol, you still have to shampoo your scalp. Once or twice a week, use Neutrogena T-Gel (or any other tar-based moisturizing shampoo) to clean and moisturize your scalp. Since you'll have no natural hair oils for a while, your scalp needs extra nourishment at this time.

A Perk: Your Sunglasses Finally Stay On.

If you're like me, you've always been annoyed that your sunglasses constantly slip down your nose, despite repeated visits to the optician to get the eyepiece screws tightened. Well, no more. If you slide them underneath the elastic band of your wig, presto! They stay on . . . until *you* decide to remove them!

Don't Remove Your Wig While Driving. It May Be Hazardous to Other Drivers.

Let's face it. While you'll eventually decide that losing your hair is a minimal inconvenience in the scheme of beating cancer, at times the wig bit becomes a nuisance. It itches, it's hot during the summer months, and the elastic can even give you headaches. You just want to yank it off. Word of warning: Be careful about when and where you do so. I was driving on a fairly deserted, country highway one summer evening on my way to visit family in Vermont. I had been in the car for a few hours, and my wig just plain itched. So, thinking that I was completely alone in the countryside, I yanked it off. However, glancing in my rearview mirror, I suddenly realized that another car had just pulled on to the road from an entrance ramp and was swerving behind me, having done a double-take from shock at seeing my hair ripped off. Apologies to the driver, wherever you may be. . . .

Ice Caps: They Only Make Your Head Feel like It's Stuck in a Snowbank.

You might hear all sorts of crazy schemes to help preserve your hair during chemotherapy. If you hear about the ice cap, a bathing cap–like piece that supposedly freezes your head so the chemotherapy drugs can't get to the hair follicles, spare yourself the time and expense of tracking one down. As my oncologist said to me, "Even if they worked, I wouldn't let you use them." You don't want to restrict blood flow to any part of the body, because you want the chemotherapy drugs to move throughout the entire body to get any stray cancer cells wherever they may be lingering. So they don't necessarily work, but do they make you feel any better? Only if you like having your head stuck in a snowbank.

An Additional Perk: You Won't Have to Shave or Wax.

While everyone is different, and the hair on your head is the most visible to the outside world, be prepared to lose all your body hair. It might happen later in the treatment cycle, or it may not happen at all, but you might get the benefit of not having to shave your legs or wax your bikini line for several months.

I Never Knew I Was So Attached to My Eyebrows and Eyelashes.

On some of the stronger chemos such as Adriamycin or Taxol, your eyebrows and eyelashes might start to thin after several treatments, and long after you've lost the hair on your head. While you've managed to accept that by now and maybe even have some fun with wigs, scarves and hats, when your eyelashes and brows start to go, you'll really begin to feel ugly. Not to worry. Go to the drugstore. Buy Maybelline eyebrow powder. It costs about $2.00. There, now you have very natural-looking eyebrows. It beats the fake-looking pencils. Stop fretting and start smiling (it will also make your eyebrows look better).

Regarding eyelashes, be careful about fakes. The glue can cause infections. So you might just play it safe and use a dark eye pencil to rim your otherwise beautiful eyes.

Keeping the Sparkle in Your Eyes

It's Time for Eyeglasses That Can Be Worn in Public.

Chemotherapy is very drying to the body overall, which means that your eyes may become drier, more sensitive, and more easily irritated than usual. If you wear contact lenses, this means that by evening—or sooner—your contacts may feel like sandpaper. Do you really want your only option to be skulking home in the privacy of your own bedroom to don those Coke-bottle eyeglasses you've had since John Travolta danced in *Saturday Night Fever*? It's time to update your eyeglass wardrobe. Get yourself a new set of spectacles that you won't be embarrassed to be seen in walking down the street. Just as you'll get accustomed to various "looks" with wigs, scarves, and hats, you might even *want* to wear your new glasses on days when your eyes are particularly irritable. What a concept!

Sunspots, Even When It's Not Sunny, Doesn't Mean You're Going Blind.

You might experience what seem like white spots, or places where your vision just seems to blank out. It's as if you're staring straight into the sun, and are temporarily blinded. If this happens, sit down, relax, and call your doctor immediately. Most likely, your *red* blood cell counts have dropped, and since these are the cells that carry oxygen throughout your body, you are not getting enough oxygen to your brain. You might just need to slow down a bit, or if it persists and if your red cells drop low enough, you might need to go to the hospital to get a blood transfusion.

Smiling with a Healthy Mouth and Teeth

Keep Your Smile Worth a Million Bucks.

Go to your dentist and get a good cleaning before you start chemotherapy. Why? Several reasons: (a) Food bacteria and particles in your teeth might cause a bad taste to develop from the drugs, and (b) you don't want to have to endure any major dental work during the course of your chemo because you will be more prone to infections. Besides, dental work is pretty miserable anytime. Why endure it now?

Fluoride the Old-fashioned Way, and Brushing a New Way.

Another tip for teeth. When you go to your dentist, make sure to ask for a bottle of fluoride. It helps keep your teeth strong and prevents cavities, which you might be more prone to due to saliva changes from the chemotherapy drugs. Also ask for a foam toothbrush, and brush with the flouride nightly before you go to bed (don't rinse it out). So this is what people did before fluorinated toothpaste!

No Flossing? Your Dentist Will Forgive You.

Your gums may become particularly sensitive, regardless of whether you develop full-blown mouth sores. And on the days your blood counts are low, you want to be careful to prevent infection or gum bleeding which might have difficulty clotting (if your platelets are low). So, make sure you use a soft-bristled toothbrush, brush frequently, but very gently, and skip the dental floss on these days. Also, avoid commercial mouthwashes, which can be irritating to your mouth.

Here's Yet Another Use for Arm & Hammer Baking Soda.

Fill up a plastic container of warm water and 1–2 teaspoons of Arm & Hammer baking soda. Keep it in your refrigerator for a few days after chemo. Rinse your mouth and gargle with it 4–5 times a day. In cooking, baking soda is the ingredient that makes things rise and puff, but in chemo, it prevents and reduces swollen, puffy gums, mouth, and throat sores. These are more an annoyance than anything else. You just don't need them.

Anything but the Metallic Flavor, Please.

You might experience strange tastes in your mouth that are indescribable, tastes that you never knew your mouth could produce. About the most positive word that can be used to describe them is "metallic," as if someone was forcing you to chew on an aluminum soda can. Don't despair; they're easily gotten rid of. I relied on mint-flavored candies (e.g., Wintergreen Life Savers or Altoids) to alleviate the taste. Other women I've spoken to have found other tastes that help, such as cinnamon (e.g., Dentyne gum) or the "sour" taste of lemon (e.g., lemon drop candies, lemon sorbet), and some even recommend chewable zinc tablets (but only on a full stomach, as they can cause nausea otherwise). Alternatively, if you aren't experiencing nausea or mouth sores, try foods with strong flavors such as Mexican or Indian. Find what works for you and stick to it.

Slippery Elm Isn't a Tree Bark. It's a Throat Lozenge. And Lysine Isn't a Household Cleaner.

There sure are some strangely named items in health food stores. But if you have the courage to insert anything named slippery elm into your mouth, you deserve some relief. You'll be pleasantly surprised to learn that slippery elm throat lozenges can relieve the sore throats associated with chemotherapy. Alternatively, lysine is an amino acid also found in health food stores that can counter mouth sores and is taken in pill form daily.

Gentleness: Disguising Foods for Your Finicky Mouth.

If you do develop mouth sores during the course of treatment, you will face additional challenges to maintain the good nutrition your body needs right now. Since your mouth is so sensitive, it will be a very finicky gatekeeper as to which foods it will allow you to swallow. Think gentleness—yes, any means by which you can make your foods gentler or easier to get down will be greatly appreciated by your tender mouth. A few examples include: avoid acidic, spicy, or salty foods; eat foods pureed, stewed, or otherwise soft in texture; and moisten dry foods with sauces or liquids. Sounds a bit bland? Well, yes, but the good news is that these types of foods will also be best to manage any nausea. Your mouth and your stomach have joined efforts in their conspiracy against you.

Ask Your Doctor for Magic Mouthwash.

If none of these milder remedies seem to work for you, ask your doctor for a prescription for "magic mouthwash," which is ⅓ viscous lidocaine, ⅓ Benadryl elixir, and ⅓ Maalox or Mylanta. Doesn't sound like something that tastes wonderful, so it must help alleviate and heal those bothersome mouth sores.

Skin Radiance, Not Pallor

The Magic Ingredient of Beautiful Skin? Moisture (and No, This Is Not a Beauty Ad).

Since we now know that chemo is both very drying, and that it kills rapidly growing cells in the body, we might anticipate that it can wreak havoc on your skin. Yes, it might. As the protective layer of your body, your skin is under constant assault by the environment and, therefore, in a continual cycle of expending energy to renew itself. And moisture is the magic ingredient to aid in that renewal process. So, when chemo dries out your skin, your body has to work harder to replace skin cells, and the last thing your body needs right now is to work any harder on anything that's not related to healing. So moisturize your skin at least twice daily to avoid dryness. This is doubly important, since dry skin can also be itchy, and you don't want to be annoyed with scratching that might open the skin to infection in your immunocompromised state. A few hints:

- *Use moisturizers made for "sensitive skin."* Your skin might be more sensitive now than usual, so save those perfumed body creams.
- *Pat dry, don't rub.* When you get out of the shower, don't rub with a rough towel. Rubbing removes the top layer of skin, which may make it more susceptible to irritation. Instead pat gently, which leaves skin damp but not dry, and immediately moisturize.
- *Try petroleum jelly or mineral oil as your safest bet.* If your skin is too irritated for moisturizer right now, try these as an alternative. There is absolutely nothing in either product to irritate your skin. For easiest application (so they don't go on too goopy), try smoothing on a thin layer as soon as you step out of the shower. Wait a minute or two and then use an old T-shirt or other cotton cloth to pat yourself dry and absorb any excess (but leaving moisture to soak into your skin).
- *Don't overshower.* Wetting the skin is a vicious cycle. You want to add moisture to your skin by trapping it under the moisturizer, but you don't want to strip away moisture. Keep your showers short and at lukewarm temperature.

Rashes: Report Them to Your Doctor Immediately. Do Not Pass Go.

Consider your skin a reflection of what's going on inside your body. So, when a skin rash appears—be it itchy and hive-like or raw and tender—interpret it as a glaring beacon from your body that something may have gone awry. Therefore, if you ever get a rash, no matter how small or insignificant you think it is, report it to your doctor immediately. Given that your body is being exposed to many variables right now, a rash can signal many things, including a drug reaction to one or a combination of your chemotherapy drugs, or an infection acquired when your white blood counts dropped too low. In some situations, your doctor might even decide to biopsy your rash to determine if you'll be able to tolerate certain drugs in the future.

Sun Is Your Enemy. Umbrellas Are Your Friends.

Regardless of whether you have been a sun worshipper or sun avoider to date, now is the time to believe that pale skin is beautiful. Avoid the sun at all costs for several reasons. First, chemotherapy can make you photosensitive, which means your skin's sensitivity to sunlight is dramatically increased (just like when you take antibiotics, if you've ever experienced that). Not only can you get severe sunburns, but you also risk rashes and inflammation of the skin (neither of which you need right now in your immuno-suppressed state). Second, a bad sunburn will also put your arm at risk for lymphedema if you had lymph nodes removed. And if that's not enough, a sunburn takes a toll on your body, which must use energy to repair the damaged skin, just like dry skin. So, wear sunscreen whenever you are outside. Wear double your normal SPF, and make sure it protects against both UVA and UVB rays, not just UVB. A few brands to try are: Shade, Pre-Sun, Ombrelle, or Neutrogena. And carry an umbrella with you, even on sunny days. Use that umbrella, or seek out shade whenever possible.

Now Is Not the Time to be a Beach Bum. Cover Up and Catch the Sunset.

If you are going through treatment during the summer as I did, going to the beach can be very good for your mental state. But make sure you cover up, not only with sunscreen, but with tightly knit cotton clothes (most summer clothes are loosely woven for breatha-bility) and with a wide-brimmed hat. And limit your time there. I found that I also became very weak and even dizzy if I spent more than 15 or 20 minutes at a time in intense sunlight. Go late in the day, near sunset when the sun is less intense. It's beautiful then, and you'll better be able to enjoy and appreciate every minute of it.

Pigment Changes May Be Nature's Attempt at a Tattoo.

The bad news: During treatment, you may notice spotty pigment changes in your skin. The good news: Any discoloration should fade once treatment is completed. If you notice brown, gray, or bluish patching or streaks, there is nothing you can do right now. During chemotherapy, chemicals may deposit in the skin, but these will eventually fade. Alternatively, if you notice spontaneous bruising or bruise-like reactions, get them checked immediately. This might signal that your platelet count is too low and you may need a blood transfusion.

Nail Changes: Any Excuse for a Manicure (and Pedicure).

Technically, your nails are part of your skin, and can be affected by chemotherapy in several ways. First, since your body is using energy to heal, any energy used to grow nails might be temporarily diverted. So, your nails may decide to grow in spurts, starting and stopping, which can produce either grooves across your nail horizontally (these are called beau's lines), or even vertical ridges. Second, the kind of pigment change discussed above might also affect your nails in the form of horizontal bands of discoloration. Both symptoms are absolutely harmless, but why have one more visual reminder that your body has been violated? The remedy? All can easily be disguised by a good manicure, including buffing, polishing, plus a strong alpha-hydroxy moisturizer used nightly. Two to try are Vasoline Hand & Nail Cream and Eucerin Plus. Any excuse for a manicure (but don't clip the cuticles)!

Treat Yourself to a Makeover ... Compliments of Your Cancer.

Managing the side effects of chemotherapy is just as much about psychological as well as physical stamina. At some point, you might begin to feel just plain ugly. Perhaps it's because you are a bit pale and weak from treatment, because you've lost your eyelashes and eyebrows, or just because you've been avoiding the sun. Don't fret. Feeling pretty again is just one phone call away. The American Cancer Society sponsors a complimentary makeover program called "Look Good, Feel Better." Offered monthly, these 2-hour group sessions lead you through a 12-step program to give your looks (and spirits) a lift. Plus, you are given a box full of cosmetics specific to your skin type and color to take home, compliments of leading cosmetic companies (Estée Lauder, Chanel, Lancôme, etc.). You're even provided with a basic wig if you need it. For details, call 1-800-395-LOOK or your local American Cancer Society office (see page 41).

Walking: A Better Alternative to Being Asked If You Have Jaundice.

One of the most frequent and visible side effects of any chemotherapy treatment (besides hair loss, which can be hidden) is a pale, sallow complexion. However, there is a very easy way to combat this ghost-like pallor, and no experience or expense is required: walking. A daily walk—as brisk as you can muster—in fresh, crisp air is good for your circulation, and will help restore color to your cheeks. It also will help keep your head clear, and help prevent weight gain from drugs or your currently more sedentary lifestyle.

Solving the Mysteries of Your Appetite: Nausea, Your Digestive System, and Nutritional Needs

Mint Will Become Your Favorite Flavor.

Despite what the chemo nurses do with new "wonder drugs" to mitigate any nausea you might experience, your stomach may turn some loops at some point during the course of your treatment. Drink mint tea (chamomille or ginger work too) to settle your upset stomach. Suck on mint candies—Life Savers, Tic Tacs, or Altoids— to get rid of the rancid taste in your mouth. Drink mint-flavored Phillips' Milk of Magnesia to get you going at the other end. And yes, you'll know when you need it.

Animals Are Friendlier.

Buy a big jar of animal crackers. Leave them out on your kitchen counter in view. Eat them rather than saltines—the old standby—to settle your nausea. Why? They're cute. They'll make you smile.

Trick Your Finicky Stomach into Accepting Some Food.

You might experience the rare sensation that you just don't want to eat, because everything you look at makes your finicky stomach turn somersaults. (Why can't I borrow some of this when I'm trying to diet?) Well, here are a few ways to "trick" your stomach into wanting food, so you can get the nutrients you need to maintain your strength:

- *Do eat:* Bland foods, room-temperature foods, smaller portions more frequently, soft foods (e.g., mashed potatoes, yogurt, rice, cooked eggs), pureed or stewed foods, breads before other foods, noncarbonated drinks (best to settle an upset stomach is "flat" lukewarm ginger ale or ginger tea).
- *Don't eat:* Spicy, fatty, or greasy foods; extremely hot or cold foods; foods with strong odors; big meals; sweets; or alcohol.

Staying Hydrated: Eat Foods That also Provide Fluids.

If you experience nausea and vomiting for more than a few hours, you'll need to find ways to prevent dehydration, something you don't need now, especially given all the chemicals circulating through your body. If you have a hard time keeping even water down, a few foods to try that both settle your stomach and provide some hydration include bananas, potatoes, apples without skins, and peas without skins.

There's Always the BRAT Diet (plus Fluids).

If you are experiencing severe problems with your gastrointestinal system—either nausea or diarrhea—you can always resort to the time-tested BRAT diet—bananas, rice, applesauce, and toast—until your system regains equilibrium. Following BRAT, plus forcing yourself to take in a lot of fluids, should make you feel better within a day or so. For fluids, try diluted fruit juices, ginger ale, or even ginger tea (slices of raw ginger root steeped in boiling water). Note that ginger has been around since ancient times as an antinausea remedy, so it must have some efficacy.

Getting Enough Fiber: Soon You'll Start Spitting Watermelon Seeds.

You might find that you need extra amounts of fiber to keep your digestive system regular. You might become constipated for a few days in each treatment cycle, more due to the antinausea drugs than chemo itself. Well, instead of Metamucil or Ex-Lax, or some other terrible-tasting product, try watermelon. It's refreshing, tastes good, provides lots of fiber, and you'll even get good at spitting those little seeds. Not as much fun, but just as effective are pineapple, kiwi, prunes, apricots, and high-fiber foods such as bran, nuts, and popcorn. Also, try sipping on refreshing lemon water. And if all else fails, ask for a stool softener.

Another benefit of exercise: It can help keep your digestive system moving.

Helping Your Immune System Fight Harder: Special Nutritional Needs during Chemotherapy.

Any woman who wants to maintain optimum health—be it pre-, during, or postcancer—should eat a well-balanced, nutritionally sound diet (See Chapter 9, "Nutrition"). However, depending on the types and severity of side effects that you experience during treatment, you may wish to consult with a dietitian or nutritionist to determine what you can do from a nutritional standpoint. For example, if you are losing or gaining weight from chemotherapy, you might alter your daily caloric intake, or rebalance the proportion of carbohydrates, fats, and protein. Or if your blood counts drop substantially, you might increase your protein intake to help keep your immune system strong, as well as to help preserve muscle tissue if you are experiencing any weakness or fatigue. Besides increasing the amount of protein, you might also broaden the types of proteins you eat, and perhaps include a bit more red meat to boost your hemoglobin levels (which are part of the red blood cells that carry oxygen through your body). Before making any dietary changes, consult with the appropriate professionals where you are receiving treatment. Your oncologist might even recommend it to you before you need to ask.

Split Opinions: Vitamins through Food versus Vitamins by Pills.

A special note on vitamins, herbs, or any type of nutritional supplements. If you are taking any form of supplement, or are considering beginning a program to help you manage the side effects of chemo, be sure to tell your oncologist. Some doctors prefer that you not take anything during your treatment, as supplements may interfere with the effectiveness of the drugs. My oncologist is so against supplements that he believes, "If God meant for people to take vitamins, he would have grown those little pills on trees! Get your vitamins through food!" However, others will not be concerned if you take a daily multivitamin or other basic supplements. Once you are finished with treatment, you can follow whatever nutritional program you believe works for you (see Chapter 9, "Nutrition," for a discussion of basic nutritional needs for cancer survivors).

Eating Cautiously to Avoid Infection: Because Food Poisoning Is Never Fun, Especially Not Now.

Since you may be immune-compromised throughout your treatment (especially on those days of your cycle when your white counts dip down), you'll want to take extra caution during this time to ensure that you don't eat any foods that could give you an infection or food poisoning. If you do, your body may not be able to fight it on its own, requiring antibiotics to get rid of it, and most likely a delay in your treatment until you're well again. So, since food poisoning is never fun, especially not now, a few easy ways to avoid the risks:

- *Fruits and vegetables.* Stick to fruits that can be peeled (e.g., oranges, melons, bananas) and vegetables that can be peeled (e.g., sweet potatoes) or cooked (e.g., broccoli). Avoid hard-to-clean raw fruits (e.g., berries, grapes), or raw vegetables (e.g., celery, lettuce), unless you have a good produce cleanser (which can be found at health food stores), or simply wash well with a bit of dish soap and water.

- *Meats.* Stick to meats that are cooked well, and avoid sushi or anything else raw.
- *Dairy products.* Because of the pasteurization standards in our country, dairy products like milk and yogurt are fine (just check the expiration date). However, be wary of any foods prepared with mayonnaise, which could spoil (e.g., potato salad, coleslaw, pasta salad with mayonnaise dressing), especially in warm weather.

And a special caution for restaurant dining: Eat only cooked foods. Since you don't know how the food was washed, handled, or prepared, skip the uncooked items such as salads, sushi, or milk-based products, etc.

Befriend Taxicab Drivers. It May Become a Lifelong Affair.

If you live in a major urban area where taxicabs are a primary mode of transportation (e.g., New York, London, Chicago), be nice to your cab drivers and you'll receive VIP treatment. Since most mere mortals feel nauseous in the backseat of cabs on a good day, here's how to transform your public transportation experience to survive those months of chemotherapy.

When the cab pulls over to pick you up, instead of jumping in the back and barking directions, knock on the front window of the passenger side. Very sweetly and politely tell the driver that you are not feeling quite well, and in fact are about to vomit, and you'd greatly appreciate it if you could sit in the front seat next to him. After a look of complete astonishment and all the blood draining from his face, he'll grumble, "Okay." Jump in and enjoy yourself. You won't get sick. It's much cooler in the front. And passersby will give you funny looks. Maybe this should continue indefinitely.

Tracking and Maintaining Blood Count Levels

A NOTE FROM THE DOCTOR

R̥ *The Delicate Dance of Blood Cells and Chemotherapy*

Earlier we discussed the "toxicity," or deadliness, of chemotherapy to many types of rapidly dividing cells in your body. But perhaps the most important toxicity to monitor is to the bone marrow. Your bone marrow makes three types of cells, each with a critical function in your body. Red cells carry oxygen throughout your body to tissues. Platelets help your blood to clot when you cut yourself. And as part of your immune system, white cells fight infection.

The destruction of these three cell types makes your body vulnerable to a range of situations that require immediate medical attention. If your red cell count (equivalent to "hemoglobin") drops, you may become weak or short of breath, and in extreme cases may require a blood transfusion to get enough oxygen circulating through your body. Low platelet counts may predispose you to excessive bleeding or bruising. If the platelet counts drop too low, these may also be transfused. And finally, white blood cells are the most likely to decline after chemotherapy because they live for a shorter period than the other types. Unfortunately, there are no white cell infusions available. So, during the lowest white blood cell count days of your chemo cycle, you would need to be hospitalized for any fever, or perhaps even a cold, because infections at this time can be life-threatening. If you get a fever, call your doctor immediately. You'll be fine, but you might just end up in the hospital on antibiotics for a few days, under the watchful eyes of your doctors.

Neupogen™ at Night Keeps White Blood Cells in Sight.

If you are receiving one of the chemotherapy regimens that is more toxic to your blood cells, your doctor might recommend a CSF, or "colony-stimulating factor," to stimulate your bone marrow to replenish white blood cells more quickly. Theoretically, the less time that your counts are low, the less time you are susceptible to serious infection. Neulasta, made by Amgen, is the most commonly used one, although there are others. Amgen also makes Neupogen, a short-acting version of Neulasta, and Genzyme makes Leukine, a similar product that some doctors prefer. Talk to your oncologist about which CSF is best for you.

After a shot, you might experience some mild side effects, such as bone pain, a slight fever, or redness at the injection site. Call your doctor to discuss any symptoms. Tylenol is often used to mitigate any discomfort.

Pay Attention to Cravings and Changes in Energy Patterns. Your Blood Cells Are Talking to You.

Ever heard the expression, "I'm so hungry, I could eat a cow?" It must have come from someone undergoing chemo whose red blood counts were low. When your body is low on red blood cells and therefore oxygen, as well as iron and other essential nutrients, you may experience cravings for foods high in protein and iron, such as red meat. So, go ahead, it's okay to eat that cow (even if you are otherwise a vegetarian). Other foods that will nourish your body through this deficit include liver or any organ meat, raisins, split peas, grains, and legumes.

98.6°F? 100.5°F? Know Your Doctor's Magic Numbers.

One key indicator as to how your body is being affected by chemotherapy is your temperature. You will probably take your temperature more times during your treatment period than you have in your entire life to date. Since the chemotherapy may destroy white blood cells that are the basis of your immune system, you will be more susceptible to infections than normal. If you feel at all warm, take your temperature immediately. But unless it reaches a threshold level that your doctors indicate (mine was 100.5°F degrees Fahrenheit), don't worry. Most people have minor daily fluctuations around 98.6°F. I even discovered that my "normal" body temperature is closer to 98.0°F. However, on several occasions my temperature rose to 99.2°F or 99.4°F. The first time it happened, I was terrified that the thermometer was headed straight up to 100.5°F+ and I to the quarantine unit of the hospital. But I learned to calm down, become less anxious, and dismiss a minor fever as a "normal" reaction of my body to chemotherapy.

If you do get a fever that reaches your doctor's threshold number, call your doctor immediately (see "Eleven Reasons to Call the Doctor," page 140). You might have an infection and need to go to the hospital for antibiotics to help fight it. If your temperature is below that "threshold" but you feel lousy, you should still call.

The Pharmacy Might Run Out of Thermometers.

You don't need to invest in fancy, electronic or digital thermometers to monitor your temperature. The old-fashioned glass types that cost $3.00 are just fine, and according to some nurses, the most accurate of all. Buy several and keep them in a variety of places— your home, office, car, purse, etc. Then, whenever you feel warm, you'll always have one within arm's reach. (Hey, isn't that Coca-Cola's tag line?)

Do Your Fingers Feel like a Pincushion?

By the end of your treatment, you will have been poked, prodded, and pricked with so many needles that you might feel like you've turned into one of those cherry-tomato pincushions. I had my fingers stuck nearly three times per week to monitor the effect of the chemotherapy on my blood counts. The secret to not becoming a pincushion? Lots of moisturizer or petroleum jelly. By keeping your hands very moisturized, and even coating them with Vaseline at bedtime each night, your skin will stay soft, and won't become tough, irritated, or so callous that it is difficult to insert needles without discomfort.

Develop a Handwashing Fetish . . . at Least Temporarily.

The simplest way to acquire and pass along germs and bacteria is with your hands. So, a little extra care, even obsession, right now in practicing good hygiene will go a long way in avoiding picking up unnecessary germs. Wash your hands several times a day with an antibacterial cleanser. Also don't cut or tear cuticles (which you should never do again in order to prevent lymphedema), and clean any scrapes, cuts, or open sores immediately with a topical antibiotic ointment.

Avoiding Infections: Now Is Not the Time to Frequent Concert Halls.

By now, you might think I'm paranoid about immunosuppression and susceptibility to infections, but just to be extra conservative, I also felt more comfortable avoiding places and people during treatment that could have made me vulnerable. I decided not to frequent crowded, indoor spaces, such as movie theaters, concert halls, and airplanes (your doctors probably won't let you fly given both the germs in recirculated airplane air, and the need to be close to your medical facility should you develop an infection). And if you can avoid it, you might also stay away from large concentrations of children, such as schools, as kids are notorious germ-carriers. Your doctors will have varying opinions on this, as some claim that you are more likely to get an infection from within your body than from external sources, but at least I felt I was protecting myself as much as I could. Otherwise, what's the use of all that extra hygiene?

Understanding Menopausal Symptoms: The Real Thing?

Brace Yourself for a Wild Estrogen Ride . . .

From our discussion of the theory of chemotherapy, you now understand that chemotherapy agents can damage ovaries, since they contain some of the fastest-growing cells in the body. If chemo does damage, it will potentially reduce the amount of estrogen circulating in your body, as your ovaries produce estrogen. This can cause menopausal symptoms such as hot flashes, vaginal dryness, and even mood swings. Such symptoms may be temporary and disappear after you finish treatment, or you may actually experience premature menopause. The closer you are to menopause—say past age 40—the more likely it will be triggered now. However, no doctor will be willing to quote you statistical probabilities for your age group, since this entire subject has not yet been extensively studied. There are just some things that must be left to fate . . . and besides, when the choice is your life or potentially your fertility, it quickly gets put in perspective.

. . . And New Surprises at "That Time of the Month."

Whether you've had regular menstrual cycles or problematic, irregular periods, you've probably never eagerly awaited "that time of the month." Well, prepare yourself for chemotherapy to add another variable to the monthly mystery. You may experience a wide range of changes in your cycle, including irregular or absence of periods, changes in bleeding patterns, increased cramps—or simply no changes at all. Whatever happens, there's not much you can do except wait it out. When you're through treatment, if you still have irregularities or symptoms that bother you, talk to your gynecologist about alternatives for getting you back on an even keel, and possibly other tests to determine that changes in menstrual patterns do not represent new gynecological conditions.

A Terrifying Thought: Hair Comes Back. Fertility Doesn't.

Perhaps the scariest aspect of this entire ordeal, if you are a woman of childbearing years, is the risk of premature menopause. For me, someone who had always wanted four children in her life, this was almost more terrifying than the cancer. It strikes at the core of your being. Yes, losing your hair is scary because it's the most visible. But the infertility risk punches you in the gut. If you're in my situation, and haven't had your children yet because Prince Charming hasn't appeared at your door, the emotions become even more complicated. You doubt that any man would ever want to marry you if you can't have his children. Even if you do have a partner, you wonder if he'll still find you attractive if the essence of your womanhood is gone. So what to do? Okay, take a moment and pity yourself. Admit that this is a terrifying uncertainty. Then go visit your grandparents (or borrow someone else's). Look at how much your grandfather still adores your grandma. She's been through menopause and she still has men chasing after her! (For more on fertility and children after breast cancer, see Chapter 8, "Longer-Term Issues: The Aftermath").

Cooling Agents for Hot Flashes.

If severe enough, hot flashes may be the toughest menopausal symptom to deal with for several reasons. Not only are they uncomfortable, unpredictable, and socially embarrassing, but they can also disrupt sleep patterns, causing irritability and potentially mood swings. If you have hot flashes that significantly bother you, discuss the problem with your oncologist or gynecologist, as there are medications that can provide some relief. However, there are also homeopathic and nutritional remedies that seem to ease the discomfort. Foods that provide estrogen-like substances from plants, called phytoestrogens, such as soy and tofu, can minimize hot flashes, as well as provide important cancer-fighting properties. Again, discuss any alternative therapy with your doctor, as extreme amounts or certain herbal remedies can be dangerous. (See Chapter 9, "Nutrition," for a discussion of the potential role of soy in fighting breast cancer.)

Some women find that 800 milligrams of vitamin E is helpful. If not, some classically used antidepressants, such as Effexor and Prozac, can be of enormous benefit. Effexor, for example, is helpful at merely one third the lowest dose used for depression. Discuss the use of these medications with your physician.

No Sex? Boy, I Must Be Really Sick!

You wouldn't be "normal" if you didn't experience some sort of variation in your sexual appetite during treatment. Your body is experiencing an incredible number of complex, interrelated changes

—hormonal estrogen changes, the psychological trauma of the experience, physical discomfort from surgery, fatigue, etc. So, sex may or may not be at the top of your priority list right now. Don't beat yourself up, or let your partner make you feel guilty if it isn't. Also, you never know what will happen. Some women experience an increase in sexual desire, as the intensity of the cancer experience draws them closer than ever to a strong, stable, supporting, caring partner. As always, open, honest communication with your partner is key to getting through this together.

AstroGlide? Isn't That a Toy for George Jetson's Dog?

You might be lucky enough to maintain a healthy sexual appetite and physical stamina through treatment, but you experience vaginal dryness from chemotherapy or menopause-like symptoms. Just remember to use a nonhormonal (yes, hormones may fuel the growth of breast cancer cells, so stay away from them) vaginal lubricant such as AstroGlide, K-Y Jelly, or Replens. Ask your gynecologist for other suggestions or alternatives.

ERT May Be Designer Estrogen, but Survivors Shouldn't Be Fashionable.

If you're already on or considering estrogen replacement therapy (ERT) to counteract the effects of menopause, think again. Once you've been through breast cancer, the last thing your body needs is more estrogen. If you are concerned about the postmenopause, long-term health issues that ERT is intended to address—such as management of osteoporosis or heart disease—discuss alternatives with your oncologist or gynecologist.

Another indication of the rapidly advancing world of women's health: While current forms of ERT are not advisable for breast cancer survivors, there are a variety of new therapies in development that eliminate the estrogen risks.

Always the Optimist: Less Estrogen Means Less Risk (Maybe).

And in the end, if you do experience premature permanent menopause (or are already through it and now find yourself ineligible for ERT), look at the bright side. As my oncologist remarked one day when I was flipping out about potential menopause, "Hey, if you do go through menopause, it's better for your cancer!" While my cancer was theoretically gone after surgery, what he meant was the less estrogen circulating through the body, the less risk of estrogen stimulating any remaining mircoscopic cells to start replicating and cause a recurrence.

And a Few More Words . . .

"If You Have to Visit the Emergency Room, Remember That It's the Best Place You Could Be at That Time."

Most women have one goal during chemotherapy—to stay out of the hospital. However, since there's nothing you can do to control how your individual body will react to various drugs, and since the doctors have no way to tell you exactly which side effects you might experience and to what degree, you might find yourself having to visit the emergency room at some point. I did twice, to be honest. Yes, it is a very demoralizing, depressing experience to sit in the admissions area and listen to all the other types of cancer with which the people around you are consumed. However, you just have to remind yourself that at that moment in time, there is no place else you should be, that the doctors know how to handle whatever side effect you are experiencing that has gotten out of hand (e.g., fever, rashes, low blood counts), and that you are probably the healthiest person those ER doctors have seen all day. If you like, you could ask a family member or friend to accompany you to help keep you upbeat. You might also bring a good book. It might take several hours to get seen because as long as your vital signs (e.g., breathing, heart rate) are normal, you might fall behind a variety of other more urgent "emergencies." Hopefully, you'll be going home before you know it!

You Might Just Get Plain Ol' Sick. Remember That?

At some point during the course of your treatments, you might feel plain lousy. And the first thing you will do is blame it on the chemotherapy, or panic that your unusual ache or pain means that the cancer has recurred and metastisized throughout your body. But remember, chemotherapy temporarily suppresses your immune system, so you are more susceptible to any colds, flus, or viruses going around right now. Relax, you might just be plain old sick. (But if you do have unusual pains in your bones or joints that last more than a couple weeks, do mention them to your doctor.)

Will My Body Ever Be Normal Again?!?!

Yes, it will, in just a few short months. About halfway into the treatment phase, you might reach this exasperated state. Once you've been through a few cycles, the initial trauma and fear of chemotherapy are behind you, so you can anticipate and manage treatments. However, you may find that you've forgotten what it's like not to spend some portion of your day worrying about a bodily function or part—blood counts, nausea, fatigue, mouth sores, no eyelashes, bald spots, or whatever else. Just as time doesn't stand still, treatment *will* end. Persevere, and hang on by thinking about what you will be doing *next* year at this same time.

MANAGING THE PROCESS OF RADIATION TREATMENTS

If chemotherapy tests your mental and physical fortitude in getting through the cancer experience, radiation, in a strange way, has almost the opposite effect. Chemotherapy clearly reminds you that you're sick by making you feel miserable when you may have been feeling great. Yet, with radiation, you wonder if something as simple as X rays can really eradicate cancer from your body. After enduring chemotherapy (and not all of you will have experienced this), you're convinced that you must suffer more for the treatment to be really effective. Relax, it's generally not that bad, other than some skin irritation and possibly some fatigue and emotional impact. Similar to the chemotherapy section, this section will offer guidance on managing both the process of radiation treatments, as well as the physical side effects.

5-7-35: A Football Play, or Your Treatment Cycle?

While keeping track of where you were in your chemo cycles might have been confusing, radiation keeps it simple. Every day. Yes, about four weeks after surgery (or chemo), you will receive radiation on a five-day per week schedule, Monday to Friday, and generally for a duration of six to seven weeks—determined by a variety of factors—for a total of about thirty-five treatments. The theory behind daily administration of radiation dosages is that shorter, individual treatments will cause less damage to healthy tissue, allowing it to repair fully, and ensure maximum efficacy in destroying any cancerous cells. You'll most likely receive 4,500–5,000 units of radiation, divided into dosages of approximately 180 units per day, plus a "boost" to the former tumor site at the end.

Three (Painless) Phases of the Radiation Process.

After getting through chemotherapy, radiation therapy should be fairly painless (remember it's all relative). While individual reactions to both chemo and radiation vary dramatically, most women agree that, overall, radiation is much less draining, both physically and emotionally. The most difficult part is often getting to treatment every day. In addition to this logistical inconvenience, the three phases of your radiation process will generally include the following.[3]

- *The initial consultation.* In this initial consultation with a radiation oncologist, you will discuss the radiation process and how radiation will work for your particular case, based on the radiation oncologist's review of your medical records and physical exam of the surgical area. Although administration of radiation therapy today has fairly standardized protocols, it still must be customized for each woman—based on the size and shape of her breast, tumor site, lymph node involvement, the need to avoid nearby organs (e.g., lungs, heart, other breast), any special skin considerations, any previous radiation, etc. While your radiation oncologist is the lead doctor,

3. "A Patient's Guide to Radiation Therapy," from Memorial Sloan-Kettering Cancer Center, Department of Radiation Oncology, pamphlet.

your complete radiation team may include several radiation technicians, nurses, and physicists, who will be involved in the measurement and dosage calculations.

- *The simulation setup (or prep session).* Sometimes done in conjunction with the consultation, the simulation session uses sophisticated computer modeling (along with some complex geometry) to determine the area of treatment and dosage intensity based on the shape of your breast and location of the surgical incision. A simulator is an X-ray machine that mimics the actual radiation machine. The goal is to deliver radiation dosages of uniform intensity throughout the entire breast area (or chest wall in instances of mastectomy). The simulation session may also include fitting you for a custom foam molding that supports your arm and shoulder to ensure your body is placed in the exact position each day for precise targeting of the radiation beams. You simply lie on a piece of foam that inflates around you and hardens to maintain the form after you leave it. And finally, your skin will be marked for the location of the beams, either with indelible ink or more permanent tattoos. (Whether you actually receive tattoos or small marks with indelible ink pens will depend on the philosophy of the institution at which you are being treated.) Expect the session to last a few hours.

- *The daily dosage administration.* Yes, daily. For twenty-five to thirty-five days, Monday through Friday, you will receive a daily dosage of radiation. While the actual treatment may take only one or two minutes, plan for at least thirty minutes in your daily routine. This will include waiting (sometimes machines get backed up as many people are treated on the same machine each day), getting undressed, being set up on the table in your placement mold, adjusting the machine, administering the treatment, and getting dressed again. And yes, the treatment is truly painless. The only way you'll know that you are being treated is that your technician will ask you to lie very still, then will leave the room and monitor you by closed-circuit television, and when everything is set, you might hear a click of the machine going on and then off. Yes, the whole process may get to seem laborious and endless a few weeks into it, but aren't you glad your technicians are being so cautious and precise?

A recent study from Canada indicates that in some women the same total dose of radiation may be provided in sixteen sessions—four days per week for four weeks in a row—with minimal additional side effects and the same therapeutic result. Interest is also growing in partial breast irradiation (PBI), targeting only the site of the tumor with either external or internal breast devices.

A Once-in-a-Lifetime Chance, As Always.

You may have heard that you can have radiation to a specific area of your body only once in a lifetime. For example, in determining your surgery options, you were probably told by your doctors that if you choose lumpectomy and radiation, if you ever get a recurrence you would have to have a mastectomy, as your breast could not be radiated twice. By understanding the theory of radiation, you now know why. By the time you've completed radiation, you've been given almost the maximum dosage of X rays that are safe to administer to healthy tissue over the course of a lifetime. The dosage has been aggressive enough to kill the cancer, but has enabled the healthy tissue to repair its DNA. However, further radiation would endanger healthy cells permanently, so they'd become incapable of repairing themselves.

The Radiation Paradox: Risking Cancer to Cure Cancer?

"But wait!" you'll say. "Doesn't radiation cause cancer? Look at all the innocent victims of nuclear power plant fallout, or World War II radiation exposure." Yes, in large, scattered doses, radiation is carcinogenic and can lead to mutation of genetic material that can cause cells to become cancerous. However, all radiation is not alike, and there is a tremendous difference between softer, scattered environmental radiation to your entire body versus focused, targeted, intense radiation for therapeutic purposes in a controlled environment over a concentrated time. For comparison purposes, if you were to be randomly exposed in the environment to the amount of radiation that you receive over the course of treatment, you would most likely die within forty-eight hours from a central nervous system failure. Paradoxically, it is the softer, uncontrolled radiation that is more likely to cause cancer than your treatment. In fact, the risk of a secondary cancer attributable to radiation is extremely low, less than 2 percent. Isn't this a worthwhile trade-off, compared to the 35–40 percent risk of recurrence without radiation?[4]

Radiation Technicians: They'll Brighten Your Day.

Make the technicians who administer the radiation doses to you every day into your friends. After all, you'll probably see more of them over the next six weeks than you will your other friends. Plus, the better they know you and the demands of your schedule, the more likely they will do everything they can to not keep you waiting. And they might even provide you with helpful tips on managing the side effects of radiation.

Yes, You Will be Tattooed, but You're Not Yet Ready for the Motorcycle Gang.

During your simulation session, you might be tattooed with a series of small dots to mark the borders of the radiation site so that your technicians can aim the radiation beam in precisely the same spot each day. Also, as discussed, should you ever need any other radiation in your lifetime, your future doctors will be able to identify the part of your body that has already been radiated. Just hearing the word "tattoo" provoked almost greater anxiety in me than the thought of having scars on my chest. Yet, in actuality, they are only five or six minuscule markings, no bigger than the mark of a ball point pen (yes, mine are blue), that could be easily mistaken for a birthmark (if you have navy blue birthmarks). When I pointed out one that particularly bothered me due to its visibility with an open-necked shirt, my oncologist's reply was, "If any man ever notices that, marry him!" The moral of that story? Either the tattoos really aren't a big deal, or men really aren't terribly observant. You decide.

4. *The Breast Cancer Survival Manual: A Step-by-Step Guide for the Woman with Newly Diagnosed Breast Cancer,* John Link, M.D. Henry Holt and Company, 1998, p. 79.

"The Boost" Is Much Easier Than Childhood Booster Shots.

When planning your treatment dosage and schedule, your radiation oncologist might mention the need for a "boost" at the end of your treatment. Don't get scared, as the boost is nothing as bad as those booster shots you had as a child with syringes made for giants. A boost is simply the last five to seven daily treatments of an additional 1,600 units concentrated on the original tumor site—or now scar area—rather than scattered across the entire breast area. You might be switched to a different machine that delivers electron beams to administer the boost dosage, which work in a slightly different way to penetrate and stay focused in your scar area versus traditional radiation beams. And your technicians might need to make some additional markings—indelible ink only here, no need for tattoos. However, other than that, you shouldn't notice any difference from your other treatments. Besides, when you get to the boost stage, you're almost at the end, the finish line of this marathon treatment process!

Save the Antioxidants for Later.

It seems like you can't read anything these days about either nutrition or cancer prevention without tripping over this big word, "antioxidant" (see Chapter 9, "Nutrition," for a discussion of antioxidants). You might be given friendly advice to get plenty of antioxidants during radiation (e.g., drinking lots of green tea) to cleanse the radiation out of your body. Please ignore it. Why? In short, antioxidants are elements that protect cells from damage. Since the purpose of radiation is cell damage—temporary for healthy cells, permanent for cancer—then by taking antioxidants during radiation, you might negate the intended therapeutic effect of radiation. The radiation can't do its job if your body has been pumped full of antioxidants to defend it. So postpone the high-antioxidant diet until after the treatment is finished.

Rest Assured: You Are Not Radioactive.

Don't consider it a stupid question to ask. Many women wonder if they become radioactive during treatment, and if they need to avoid children or others who might be especially susceptible. Rest assured, the radiation travels only to the affected area of your body, only during the time of treatment, and is not reflected to others. And no, you won't glow in the dark either.

Yet Another "Baseline" Mammogram . . . but Be Careful of Your Emotions.

Yes, you probably have a recent mammogram from before your surgery—perhaps the one that diagnosed your cancer. However, depending on where you are treated you may be asked to go for another about 3–4 months following radiation (if you had a lumpectomy rather than a mastectomy). Since you now have scar tissue from surgery, and since radiation may alter the density and texture of your breast tissue, either temporarily or permanently, your doctors will want to have a new baseline mammogram with which to compare all future tests for changes and variations. While this is a simple routine test, your reaction may not be so simple. Returning to your mammographer's office may surprise you by evoking some very strong emotions, especially if your cancer was detected from what was supposed to be a normal, routine mammogram, from which you'd go on to work, your errands, or whatever else was your routine that day. Just in case, you might want someone to accompany you for comfort and reassurance that this *really* is just a routine, baseline mammogram. (See Chapter 9, "Ending Treatment," for more on mammography guidelines.)

MANAGING PHYSICAL SIDE EFFECTS: LOCAL AREA ADVICE

Since radiation is a local, targeted treatment as compared to chemotherapy, the side effects tend to be much more focused and localized as well. Most women experience some type of mild to severe skin changes, either burns, irritation, or pigment changes, most usually temporary and reversible once treatment is completed. However, some women also experience a very real fatigue during this time, probably due to a combination of factors. So, this section will address how to handle skin burns and irritations, as well as fatigue and the emotional aspect of radiation.

Burns and Skin Irritation

The One Time Being Fair-Skinned Doesn't Necessarily Mean Being Burned.

As a fair-skinned, light-eyed person, I've spent my life suffering the constant plight of sunburn and don't remember ever spending a day in the sun when I didn't return home looking like the nightly special at Red Lobster. So, imagine when the technicians informed me that radiation beams were like high-intensity sunshine and could cause redness, burns, and swelling! I was absolutely convinced that I would be the only person in the history of radiation who had to stop treatment due to third-degree burns. Well, what a waste of worrying. As it turned out, I had absolutely no burning, and just some minor swelling and tenderness. The moral of the story? There is no way to tell how your skin will react to treatment. Women with darker skin may have problems, while pale-skinned women might sail right through. So, don't worry needlessly, as there is nothing you can do.

No Way, a Disadvantage to Being Large-Breasted?

In a society that worships women's breasts, I've finally discovered a potential disadvantage to being large-breasted. In general, women with more skin folds in their breast area, be it large-breasted or heavier women, may experience slightly more skin irritation. Also, mastectomy patients receiving radiation may experience greater discomfort, since the radiation is concentrated closer to the surface of the chest, due to the greater concern about a recurrence in the skin.

Encouraging Your Truly Natural Body Scent . . . of Corn Starch?

During radiation, you will not be permitted to use any soaps, deodorants, powders, lotions, perfumes, or any other substances that might either: (a) interfere with radiation beams due to certain chemical or metallic (e.g., aluminum) ingredients, or (b) contain drying ingredients such as alcohol, as radiation is already drying enough. However, if you do feel compelled to use something that can keep you feeling fresh and clean, try a little corn starch. It acts in a similar manner to baby powder, without the additives. Also, if it's summertime, be sure to stay out of chlorine pools and direct sun, which are also drying to the skin.

Your doctor may make an exception to the soap rule and allow you to use a mild hypoallergenic soap such as Neutrogena. As always, discuss it first.

Tread Lightly When Washing.

If you think that you need to wash extra well since you're not allowed to use deodorants or perfumes, think again. Since your skin is in such a weakened state, you should avoid heavy scrubbing or rubbing of the radiated area. You might even eliminate any rough washcloths, sponges, or loofahs and simply use your hands.

Vitamin A to the Rescue . . . Brought to You by Advil.

Once again, that reliable anti-inflammatory Advil comes to the rescue—fondly referred to as "Vitamin A" for those who take daily doses. Advil, or any other ibuprophen such as Nuprin or even generic versions, should help lessen any swelling, tenderness, or irritation you may be experiencing.

Biafine: The Mighty Fine Burn Cream.

You've already been cautioned not to use any creams, lotions, powders, or perfumes anywhere near the breast area that will be radiated. That's the prevailing American view; the French have a better idea. A household product in France, commonly used for burns, Biafine Wound Dressing Emulsion was developed specifically for use in conjunction with radiation therapy. Just recently, it has started being imported to the United States. You don't need a prescription for it, but it's hard to find. Befriend your local pharmacist and have him or her locate it for you. Or call the toll-free number of the U.S. distributor, Medix Pharmaceuticals Americas, Inc. at 1-888-BIAFINE (242-3463). Take advantage of the free sample they might send you, because one tube is expensive. Rub it on two to three times per day (just not within four hours before treatment) to keep your breast from looking like a bright red pomegranate! But make sure to mention to your radiation oncologist that you would like to use it.

A less expensive alternative is Aquaphor, which your radiation oncologist may have samples of. The trade-off? Aquaphor is significantly more greasy, which may make a mess of your clothing.

Homeopathic Remedies: A Strange-Sounding Bunch of Ingredients?

Women I talked to offered a variety of homeopathic remedies they swore by to relieve inflammation, tenderness, and maintain the skin condition. Whether you decide to investigate St. John's wort oil, tiger balm, or red pepper cream, first discuss it with your doctor to get his or her perspective.

Grow an Aloe Plant. And Visit It Daily.

If you've never been able to keep green things alive in your home, now is the time to try again. Since ancient times, aloe has been a soothing, healing remedy for burns. So, get an aloe plant, and twice a day break off a leaf, cut it lengthwise, and gently rub the gel-like substance on the inside on your affected skin. Don't attempt the easier route here of purchasing over-the-counter aloe gel from a pharmacy, as the packaged stuff contains a hint of alcohol, which is drying and irritating.

Wear Pima Cotton. It's As Soft As the Charmin (but Don't Squeeze It Just Yet).

We've already discussed "bra strategies" during the surgery recovery period. However, it doesn't stop there. Radiation brings a whole new round of lingerie challenges. If your skin reacts to radiation and becomes burned, inflamed, or hypersensitive, you'll find it difficult to wear any bra at all. Wear 100% cotton camisoles, tank tops, and T-shirts. Not only is cotton soft, but its breathability allows air to circulate near your skin, aiding in healing and preventing a buildup of bacteria, which could lead to infection. Pima cotton is best. Although it's more expensive, it's the softest, as soft as Charmin tissue. But don't expect to be squeezed just yet, as you'll probably still hurt.

Don't even think about attempting underwire bras yet, as they may dig into your sides and rupture your skin.

A Recall Reaction: Paying Penance for All Those Days at the Beach.

You might worry that your skin will be most irritated by radiation in those areas that have not had exposure to the sun—that skin underneath your bra or bathing suit. It seems so sensitive and underexposed. Actually, the opposite is true. Radiation may give you the most trouble on the skin that has had the most sun damage already. You might even witness a "recall reaction," that is, old burns coming back to haunt you. While it might be uncomfortable, irritated, and even discolored, the skin coloring should fade to blend with the rest of your chest when radiation is completed.

Even after your treatment ends, you will need to be extra-careful to avoid sun exposure to your radiation site. Stay covered up, or wear at least SPF15 sunscreen for years afterward; in fact, forever isn't a bad idea. You've already had a lifetime of exposure. Who needs more?

Tissue Tenderness: A Permanent State of PMS?

Thankfully no. In addition to possible burns, you might also experience tenderness and swelling of the radiated tissue on your breast. In fact, you might feel like you are in a permanent state of PMS in which the breast is extremely tender—not the type of day you want to forget your sports bra at the gym. There's not much you can do about this, except wear a more supportive bra than you had previously. The good news is that it will eventually lessen over time; for a couple of years, I experienced more tenderness in the breast that was radiated, but now there is no discernable difference.

Rib Pain or Shooting Pain Does Not Mean Your Cancer Has Metastasized.

Toward the end of radiation and shortly thereafter, I noticed that whenever I stretched or twisted at the waist, I would experience a sharp twinge of pain in my left rib cage. Additionally, on occasion I would experience fleeting, shooting pains across my breast area. Once again, I terrorized myself into a panicked state where I was sure that cancer had metastasized into my bones. If I had simply known that rib pain may occur due to tissue swelling around the radiation site, or shooting pain could be a result of the combination of surgery and radiation, it might have saved me several sleepless nights. Thankfully, in my case, the rib pain disappeared after several more months, and the shooting pains lessened in frequency.

Fatigue and Emotional Aspects

Fatigue: Physical, Emotional, or Both?

Everyone will tell you that you may experience mild to severe fatigue when undergoing radiation. Yes, I was slightly more tired than usual, but I just chalked it up to having to be at the hospital for treatment early every morning before work. Other than that I was lucky to feel great! That's not the whole story. Yes, there really is a physiological reason to be aware of signs of fatigue and be careful not to overburden your body during this period. While radiation is intended to destroy any "stray" cancer cells that weren't removed surgically, it also bombards healthy cells on a daily basis. Therefore, your body requires a lot of energy for those healthy cells to heal from the damaging effects of radiation. Additionally, the stress of organizing your life around daily treatment can be draining. And finally, since often radiation therapy is the last stage of your treatment process—after both surgery and chemotheraphy—by now you might just be exhausted, both emotionally and physically. You're almost done, but you just can't quite see that light at the end of the tunnel. Hang on . . . it's coming soon.

Mystery Fatigue: Just like a Day at the Beach.

If the whole concept of fatigue from radiation still doesn't make sense to you, just think of it as a day at the beach. Why do X rays to a small area of your body make you feel completely exhausted? The same reason lounging on a beach all day under the sun's rays can make you so tired by evening. Both radiation and direct sunlight damage your healthy cells, which your body then expends energy to repair, causing you to feel more tired than usual.

Once Again, You Can Never Drink Too Much Fluid.

I'm beginning to feel like a broken record, recommending an increased intake of fluids before and after chemotheraphy, and now as part of radiation. Fluids are essential to the body's ability to repair itself from damaging substances, be they chemicals or X rays. So be sure to drink at least 8–10 glasses of water or herbal teas daily.

A Bit of Separatism Won't Cause a Civil War.

One of the more difficult aspects of radiation, I found, was maintaining the mental fortitude necessary to deal with treatment on a daily basis. Not only is the sight of a hospital or treatment facility a daily reminder that you have been "sick" but the other patients waiting with you can really be a slap in the face. Some of them will undoubtedly be much sicker than you, and look it. Stay tough. If you must, be a bit of an elitist or separatist. Emotionally distance yourself by reminding yourself that you're there only so you can get through it and on with your life.

Avoid the "Waiting Room Syndrome" As Well.

If you do decide to strike up conversations with other patients going through radiation on your schedule, be careful. While you are likely to see the same people day after day, since you are all given a regular time slot, and some nice friendships may potentially form from undergoing this intense experience concurrently, don't drive yourself insane with the "waiting room syndrome." In other words, don't compare yourself, your condition, and your treatment protocol with what anyone else is getting. Don't assume that just because someone else is getting something that you should be, too. Avoid treatment conversation. Focus on life conversation. It's much more interesting.

Use Visualization to Transform Damage into Healing.

After pages of discussing how radiation damages cells, and the need for time to heal, I'll conclude this section with an alternative thought pattern that has helped some women maintain their emotional strength through this process. Instead of thinking about radiation X rays penetrating your body to damage cancer cells, visualize them as healing rays that you mentally direct to heal your body. Such visualization not only helps you to feel empowered and active in controlling your own healing, but sidesteps the fears that might have been ingrained into you about the risks of radiation.

BALANCING WORK

Emotional Stability from Your Job? Don't Underestimate the Importance of the Workplace.

Given that the *Wall Street Journal* reminds us daily of the chaotic state of global business today, am I crazy to claim that work can be a source of security and stability? Not at all. A study of cancer survivors by the National Coalition for Cancer Survivorship and Amgen, Inc., found that 81 percent of respondents claimed that maintaining some semblance of a "normal" work routine provided a foundation for emotional stability during the ups-and-downs of getting through cancer treatment. That's why many women feel emotionally torn. If you think you want time away from the office to focus on taking care of yourself and your treatments, but simultaneously feel this strange attachment to work, almost as a crutch to maintain normalcy, calm down. You're in good company, and you'll decide what works for you—emotionally, logistically, and financially—over time.

Balancing Work Continuity with Treatment and Recovery Time: A Few Tools to Navigate.

If you communicated with your employer appropriately upon your initial diagnosis, and you can perform the essential functions of your job (see Chapter 1, "Spreading the News"), you are now positioned well to take advantage of a wide variety of rights available to you. Don't hesitate to call on these rights to help you manage the physical, emotional, and even the purely logistical time burdens of balancing your work and treatment schedules. It's perfectly okay, and in fact expected, that you might need some extra time off right now. Two federal programs that you may rely on for assistance are the Family and Medical Leave Act of 1993 (FMLA) and the Americans with Disabilities Act of 1990 (ADA). Additionally, most states offer some type of protection or rights similar to the ADA. If interested, contact your local bar association and ask for information on state employment rights. And note that many union contracts offer employment protection.

FMLA: "Family" Includes Your Own "Serious Health Condition"

The Family and Medical Leave Act was enacted in 1993 to provide employees with the opportunity to take *unpaid* leave under certain circumstances, including "a serious health condition" that makes the employee unable to perform the essential functions of his or her position. In organizations with fifty or more employees and all public agencies, an employee is entitled to up to twelve weeks in one twelve-month period, as long as the employee worked 1,250 hours during the previous twelve months. It can be taken all at once or in smaller increments over the year, but the employee must be restored to the same or an equivalent position at the end of the leave.

To enact an FMLA-sponsored leave, you must do two things as the employee: (a) provide "sufficient" notice to your employer, ideally thirty days when the situation is "forseeable," and (b) provide medical certification of need from someone on your health care team—probably surgeon or oncologist—indicating the date the condition began and the probable duration. The doctor is **not** required to disclose the underlying diagnosis without your consent. Additionally, your employer may require a second or third opinion, but it must be obtained at their expense, not yours.

ADA: Cancer Is a Significant (Perceived) Disability

Passed in 1990, the premise of the Americans with Disabilities Act appears simple, but is, in fact, extremely complicated and open to significant interpretation. Quite simply, it serves as a national mandate to eliminate employment discrimination against individuals with disabilities in organizations with more than fifteen employees, and requires employers to provide **"reasonable accommodation for known disabilities."** However, these five simple words are loaded with meaning for cancer:

- **Disability:** Defined as "current or historical physical or mental impairment that substantially limits a major life activity" such as working. While this doesn't immediately appear to be relevant for cancer, it also includes the *perception of disability* as a result of stigmas, attitudes, or unsubstantiated myths, such as the myths of cancer in the workplace (see Chapter 1, "Spreading the News").
- **Known:** Your employer must know about your disability. Therefore, you need to carefully inform them about your needs upon initial diagnosis.
- **Reasonable accommodation:** This clause places the burden dually on the employee and the employer to determine the optimal solution. The employer's obligation is to provide a job restructuring or modified work schedule to allow for medical treatments without "undue burden" to them, defined in economic terms—an accommodation not prohibitively "costly, disruptive, or fundamentally alters the nature of the business or operation." Your obligation as the employee is to be flexible, and perhaps even offer suggestions. For example, you might schedule your chemotherapy sessions on Friday afternoons rather than midweek, if it will be less disruptive to your job. However, under the law, you aren't required to, simply to accommodate your employer, if your doctors advise otherwise.

ADA protects you not only in the near-term, during treatment, but over the long term as well, and applies to most human resource functions: hiring, assignments, leave, performance evaluations, training and benefits. This means, for example, that the fact that you were out for cancer treatment can't be held against you in a performance evaluation. So, how can you best ensure protection under ADA? Two ways. First, formally disclose to your employer that you have a disability, which hopefully you've already done upon your diagnosis to activate your rights. And second, offer suggestions of what types of accommodations will best help you. The process of identifying and providing accommodations should be interactive. Rather than fearing an adversarial relationship, use your employer as an ally or partner in your breast cancer battle.

And If Your Rights Aren't Heard, Prepare for Alternatives, but Don't Necessarily Rush into Court.

The specifics of any one situation with regard to human resource policies and employment law always involve a complex set of issues with many viewpoints as to exactly what constitutes fairness. Hopefully, you work for an organization that you respect for its integrity and values (that's why you choose to work there). However, in the rare, unfortunate situation that you feel you are being treated unfairly in the workplace, here are a few things you might do:

- *Keep meticulous records.* The minute you sense even an iota of discrimination due to your cancer, start to keep detailed notes of any suspicious incidents. How do you know? You just know. Your instinct is enough to warrant action. Get a notebook, and keep records of dates, times and places of conversations and/or actions taken, including the people involved and witnesses. Therefore, if you ever should need to exercise your legal rights in a lawsuit, you have tangible, concrete situations to put forward for consideration. (Note: *Don't* rewrite original notes, and *don't* use a computer, especially a hard drive from which data might be copied. The strongest evidence in court is your own contemporaneous notes taken at or near the time of the event in your own handwriting.)
- *Evaluate your objectives.* If you are thinking of filing a lawsuit, think carefully first about both the positive and negative implications. Lawsuits can be expensive, time consuming, emotionally draining and don't always result in a fair outcome. What is your key objective in suing and how sure are you that it will be achieved?
- *Consider direct negotiations.* Instead of a suit, consider confronting your employer directly and candidly in a nonthreatening manner. Most companies have formal policies and procedures for filing a grievance and an appointed compliance officer to negotiate such situations. You might even ask a member of your health care team, or one of your inner circle, to work with you and your employer to mediate and come up with a mutually agreeable, reasonable solution.
- *Watch your timing.* If, after assessing the situation and evalu-

ating your alternatives, you still believe you are not being granted your rights under ADA or FMLA, just watch the calendar. The timing window to file a discrimination suit with the U.S. Equal Employment Opportunity Commision (EEOC) is within 180 days of the unlawful actions. For more information on violations, call the EEOC at 1-800-669-EEOC.

Identifying Discrimination: When the Hair Comes Off, and the Wig Goes On, Attitudes Change.

We'll assume that most employers will be very humane, fair, and accommodating when you inform them you have cancer. After all, organizations are made up of people like us who have feelings, too. Some may have had brushes with cancer themselves. So, I'm hoping that 99 percent of you will never have to face discrimination. But if you do, how do you know? When it happens, it tends to be subtle, and usually driven by the financial impact on the organization. It will not be one defining moment or incident, but creep in slowly over time. A broad range of representative comments—by a variety of people, not just from your boss—might include: comments or inquiries about your future health, the high cost of insurance premiums due to people with health issues, a simple mention that you have "yet another" doctor's appointment, the indispensability of your job, and on and on. Comments may run from subtle to blatant, where one boss exclaimed, "When you're gone, we'll repaint this office." What? Does that mean gone from this office, or the big gone, the gone in the sky? You don't want to stick around that office long enough to find out. Exercise your rights. First, call your HR department in confidence to see if they can approach the individuals in possible violation. Call the EEOC for a free consultation or your state government Division of Human Rights. Furthermore, if you want an attorney's opinion, contact the local bar association, who will refer you to an "attorney referral" program in your area. A lawyer will meet with you for a minimal consultation fee to determine if you have a case and how to proceed.

A word of warning: Any of the public programs like EEOC or your State Division of Human Rights can take years to get to court. Consider if and how you really want to proceed.

And Remember, If It's Time to Make a Move, You're Now "Portable."

Job mobility for cancer survivors has increased dramatically since the passage of the Health Insurance Portability and Accountability Act of 1996, commonly known as the Kennedy-Kassebaum Act (for the sponsoring senators). As the biggest piece of health care legislation passed in the last ten years, it guarantees continuing insurance coverage for individuals with chronic conditions (e.g., cancer, organ transplants, heart disease) who change insurers due to a job change. Although there are some qualifying criteria (e.g., you must have had continuing coverage for the prior twelve months), no longer can you be denied insurance due to "preexisting conditions" if you do not have a break of greater than sixty-three days of coverage. So if it's time to find a new job for a variety of reasons—change of career and life goals, subtle discrimination, whatever—take comfort in the fact that it should be easier to make the move, once you find that dream job!

Rules of the Road for Family, Friends, and Other Participants

Those of you who can see her through the entire treatment phase will deserve your own medal of honor, as this becomes the phase that can seem like a never-ending marathon. Just when she celebrates the completion of one more treatment, she may experience something new or different that sends you both into a state of panic. Although it probably is just a common side effect of her drugs, it's all new to you. So, how do you maintain your sense of sanity through this? And better yet, how do you help her find some humor and optimism during this time? How do you help her integrate her "life schedule" and "treatment schedule"? And most important, how do you stay in for the long haul, after other initial well-wishers may have dropped by the wayside?

- **Provide more uplifting reading (and viewing) material.** The treatment phase can seem very long. Just because you brought her a terrific, inspirational book after surgery doesn't mean she's still reading it six months later. Or the day after chemotherapy, when she may not be up to reading, she'd really appreciate watching a "feel good" movie. Bring her more.

- **Help make treatment day a special occasion.** Help her transform treatment day from an ominous point on the calendar to a special outing. Spend the day with her. Have lunch together (beforehand, just in case she doesn't feel terrific afterward). Schedule a manicure, massage, or something else she likes. Help her pamper herself, a bit of distraction from the reality at hand. And after it's over, celebrate one-more-session-down, one-less-to-go.

- **Be an appointment escort.** Be available to accompany her to appointments. Anytime or anywhere, even if it's seemingly insignificant. She is already overwhelmed and feeling burdened by the logistics of this experience. Worrying about who can go with her to her many appointments just adds to the magnitude of the challenge. Relieve her of this burden, and let her know specifically that whenever she needs you, you're there. And remind her, often.

- **Help manage her life, but only under her direction.** Just because she has breast cancer doesn't mean she's stopped thinking or doing. Many people mistakenly try to take over the patient's life, assuming that she's incapable of caring for herself or making decisions. Back off. A key factor in helping her maintain emotional stability throughout this experience is the feeling that she has some sense of control over her life (because her physical health is clearly out of her control right now). If you try to take over, she'll be lost. So offer to help her in ways that clearly will help and won't be threatening. If she's physically tired and weak, offer to run errands, shop for groceries, pick up the children from school, or any other of life's daily logistical activities that can zap energy. Offer to bring over a complete dinner ready to eat on a weekly basis. Offer laundry service. And ask her what else she might need. Be helpful, not intrusive.

- **Ask about something besides blood counts.** Whenever you speak with her, the first inquiry out of your mouth doesn't need to be a request for a full rundown of her physical status. Just because she had her blood counts checked today doesn't mean she wants to repeat the results ten times. Or if she does want to, she'll tell you without having to ask. So remember that she's a person with many facets and interests to her life. Draw her out of her cancer world by asking about something more interesting than test results.

- **Become a hairstylist (for short hair only).** If she anticipates wearing a wig due to certain hair loss (from a drug like Adriamycin), help her through the process. Rather than having to be traumatized by a wig fitter or hairdresser, many women feel more comfortable having a good friend or family member cut their hair short as soon as it starts to fall out. Help her cut it short, and focus on the positive aspect of trying a new look. If you make a mistake, it doesn't matter. It'll soon fall out or be covered by a wig.

- **Find out what foods she likes or, better yet, what she can tolerate.** You might be very well intentioned by greeting her with a wonderful box of chocolates to make her feel better (who doesn't like chocolate?), but if she's lost her sweet tooth from chemotherapy, you might not be well received. Chemotherapy often wreaks havoc with taste buds, and mouth sores may limit what foods she can tolerate. So find out if there are any foods that she particularly craves, or anything she's developed an aversion to. Then, bring her something that will make her feel better.

- **Plan a date, once a week.** Give her something to look forward to, every week, other than her next doctor's appointment. Since the treatment phase can seem endless and she may not have her normal energy level to maintain a full social schedule, or even make plans, help her along. It doesn't matter what it is, something as simple as a walk in a nearby park, or bringing over a movie and dinner. As long as she doesn't have to plan it, and it's enjoyable, she'll appreciate it. You might even get together with other family members or friends and divide up responsibilities.

- **Keep those cards and letters coming.** I apologize for sounding like a broken record in stating once again how long the six to nine months of treatment can seem. The flowers sent to the hospital won't last this endurance race. You can stow away the "get well" cards, but don't spare the inspirational or funny cards and letters. She'll appreciate having something to look forward to when the mail arrives every day—and the fact that you're still thinking of her.

- **Abide by rules of energy conservation.** Given her limited energy right now, help her keep it focused on the productive and positive, on many fronts. Physically, help her with chores and errands that she doesn't savor, so she can use her energy for more pleasurable activities, maybe something as simple as a short walk every evening. Emotionally, help keep her focused on the positive aspects of her condition—that she's lucky it was caught early, that she has such a wonderful network of support. Even more important, screen her from those who expend negative energy, either fearing the worst for her in every situation, or living out their own cancer anxieties through her experience. And logistically, remind her that with every treatment, and every day that passes, she's one day closer to completing her journey through breast cancer.

PART IV

GETTING BACK TO LIFE

CHAPTER 8
Ending Treatment

Wow. You're done with treatment so it must be time to celebrate, right? Well, maybe not so enthusiastically right away. The end of treatment may require precarious navigation of an unexpected torrent of emotions from which you emerge on the other side back in your "normal" life. This chapter will cover:

- The strange emotional roller coaster of *Leaving the Comfort of Your Regimen.*
- Some information on *Follow-up Visits* with your health care team for the next five years and what to expect.
- A bit on some *Longer-term Issues* regarding bodily changes you may encounter, including advice for your routine ob-gyn visits and issues surrounding pregnancy and menopause.
- And guidance for the process of *Transitioning Back to Normal,* from a variety of perspectives.

LEAVING THE COMFORT OF YOUR REGIMEN
The Cliff Really Does Have a Safety Net.

Finishing treatment is a very strange experience. One of my doctors articulated it beautifully when he tried to comfort me by proclaiming, "There isn't a woman in the world who finishes this ordeal and doesn't at some point feel like she's falling off a cliff without a safety net." My sentiments exactly. You've just spent six, nine, even twelve months of your life at the center of a whirlwind of medical professionals. You could take comfort that at least you were actively *doing* something about your cancer, even if it was your weekly blood counts. At least someone was looking at your body every week. And then one day, you're just done, that's it. You're sent out into the world—a world of uncertainty—to live your life for hopefully another thirty, forty, even fifty years, without *doing* anything, except waiting to see if it ever comes back. Yes, it really does feel like you've unwillingly been nudged off the precipice of a cliff. But take a deep breath and forge ahead. As you'll see, the safety net really is still there.

Make a List of Your Fears. Then Disarm Them One by One.

You may need to quell any panic that you feel about ending treatment. Thrown out into the world again with no institution protecting you on a weekly basis, you'll end up convincing yourself that:

- You'll have a recurrence next year.
- You'll develop cancer in the other breast.
- You have permanent damage from treatment.
- If you eat one ounce of fat, you're asking for a recurrence.
- If you miss a day of exercise, you'll be dead next year.
- If you let your job stress get to you, you'll never last five years.
- You'll never find someone to date, and forget about marrying, since you've had breast cancer.

And the list goes on endlessly . . .

Stop terrorizing yourself. Turn this into a productive exercise. Make a list of your fears. Then verbalize them to someone in your inner circle, one by one, and agree on how to address or dismiss them.

A "Give-Me-More" Attitude Does Not Mean You're a Drug Addict in Recovery.

Remember when you were first told that you would probably be a candidate for chemotherapy? And you thought to yourself, "Oh no, just a little radiation maybe, but I don't need any of that chemo stuff, because my cancer isn't *that* bad"? And then you went through a mental transformation where you were pleading for the most aggressive treatment you could tolerate because you wanted to be confident that your cancer would never come back. Now it's time to reverse that mental spiral. It's time to make peace with yourself that your body has been given everything it needs at an optimal level to hopefully eliminate any remaining cancer cells and keep you disease-free.

Being Done May Not Mean You Feel like Celebrating (Right Away).

What if your family and friends are planning a well-intentioned celebration for you when you're all finished, but somehow you can't seem to get that excited about it? Instead, you might feel vulnerable, unstable, and unsure of yourself. It's the letdown after the performance, and many women seem to experience this sentiment to varying degrees. You've just expended so much emotional energy, and had to muster so much mental fortitude to get yourself through the physical stage of your cancer journey—when you couldn't afford a letdown—that now it may be time to fall apart a little. Our most primitive fight-or-flight survival instincts have kept us fighting until now, just to make sure we'd survive. But now, with the intensity of the battle over, give yourself some time to get closure on your experience, to withdraw, to grieve the loss of immortality (or at least the perceived loss, as nobody is immortal). Regroup, get ready to move on with your life. And then celebrate.

It's Time for Something Good to Happen to Me.

And one of your other sentiments, a well-deserved and productive use of mental energy, may be, "Okay, I've been through enough hell. I've had my share of catastrophe. Now it's time for something good to happen to me!" With a renewed perspective, and a crystallization of what's important to you, it's time to seek out and thrive on the positive aspects of your life.

FIVE YEAR FOLLOW-UP VISITS: WHAT TO EXPECT

Five-Year, Ten-Year Survival? Isn't Every Year a Reason to Celebrate?

You will hear a lot of discussion and read a lot about five- and ten-year survival rates. In truth, there is really no magic to these numbers, other than the doctors chose them to measure statistics in tracking the health of women survivors. The good news about the five-year mark is that the statistics show extremely high survival rates for early-stage cancer. And just to make sure you get there, you will be part of an extremely rigorous follow-up program.

You Might Not Feel It, but the Safety Net Really Is Still There.

Even though you may feel like you've been cast out unprotected into the cold world of uncertainty following your treatment phase, your doctors really haven't let you go that far. For at least the next five years your health care team will watch you like a hawk. While every hospital or medical institution will have its own variation, there are a few general guidelines that you can probably count on:

- *You'll never be more than ten to twelve weeks away from a checkup by somebody.* Several members of your team—most likely your surgeon, oncologist, and radiation oncologist—will each want to see you every four to six months for at least the next three years, and then probably semiannually for the next two years after that. If you space out your visits to each of them appropriately, you will never go more than eight to ten weeks between appointments, where at least one of them will be giving you a physical exam and a blood test.
- *You'll have an annual mammogram (and possibly sono- gram).* Regardless of your age, you will now probably be asked to go for a mammogram every year. And since mammograms do not necessarily reveal all lumps or cysts (remember, I found

my lump three months after my first baseline mammogram), you might also have a sonogram at the same time. Sonograms use ultrasound to create high-frequency sound waves that actually can distinguish between fluid-filled cysts (which absorb sound) and solid masses, either malignant or benign (that reflect sound). Consider the sonograms an extra level of security, but only if your doctor thinks they're necessary for you.

- *You may have annual bone scans and chest X rays.* Depending on your age and the extent of your original cancer, you might have an annual chest X ray or bone scan for the next five years.
- *Your ob-gyn exams will be more comprehensive.* Since anyone who has survived breast cancer is now at slightly higher risk for other "female" gynecological cancers, you should discuss with your gynecologist options for more comprehensive monitoring. This might mean more frequent visits, or even vaginal sonograms on an annual basis (more on this shortly).

And Just When You Think It's All Over, It's Really Not. The Emotions May Fade, but They Never Quite Go Away.

Be prepared for your first visit back to your oncologist's office. By this I mean not just all the normal "stuff" discussed earlier like taking notes, preparing a list of questions, and other means to monitor your health and make informed decisions. Be prepared mentally. I sure wasn't. I thought nothing of it—just a quick doctor's appointment on my way to work that morning. However, the minute I stepped off the elevator, and saw the friendly receptionist who had greeted me several times a week throughout my treatment, and then glanced past her to the blood-drawing clinic where I'd routinely had my fingers poked until they were raw, I freaked out. The world started spinning around me, I became light-headed, and all those horrible memories came flooding back to me, an instant replay of a nightmare in which I had played the starring role just six months earlier. Then I headed for the ladies' room, the same one I had used during my chemotherapy treatments (which would make me extremely nauseous six to eight hours later), and I became violently nauseous. I had to leave immediately. The mind holds an in-

credible power of association. The memories you think you've eradicated are still there, buried beneath the "normal" life that you've
returned to. Since you will never be able to predict what may trigger
a rush of memories or emotions, make sure to take someone with
you—someone to distract you from worry, someone to comfort you
if you have a tough time, and someone who will reassure you that
each time you do this from now on, it will get easier because those
memories will fade and your five-year survival anniversary is just
that much closer. Bring someone with you, always.

A Mammogram Will Never Be the Same Again: Tips for Top-Quality Care.

Whether your cancer was discovered by mammogram or not,
your future mammography experiences will most likely be extremely anxiety-provoking, even dreaded. You've had a brush with
mortality and the mammogram is theoretically a crystal ball that
provides the focus. You might ask yourself, "Oh no, what if an ab-
normality appears?" or "Worse yet, what if the films miss something?" You no longer trust yourself or the entire mammography
process. You also aren't quite sure how all the treatment you've
had—be it radiation, mastectomy, reconstructive surgery, etc.—will
affect the process and results of your mammograms. You might be
asked for multiple images in one area, or images of the chest wall if
you've had a mastectomy. Don't panic, as these are just extra precautions for thoroughness.

So how do you eliminate the panic and regain the trust?
Become an informed consumer and demand the best. There are a
few issues you should be aware to give yourself the comfort that
you are receiving the highest-quality, standard-setting mammography care:

- *The radiologist.* A radiologist is a doctor who specializes in di-
  agnostic imaging and interpreting film images such as X rays,
  MRIs, or mammograms to detect disease. All radiologists
  should be certified by the American College of Radiology, and
  adhere to the Mammography Quality Standards Act of 1992
  (which enforces *minimum* quality standards, but does not
  guarantee the highest quality). Additionally, be sure to seek

out a radiologist who specializes in breast imaging (i.e., mammography and ultrasound). By the sheer volume of films reviewed, a specialist's eye is finely tuned to perceive variations that a generalist's may not be. Moreover, a lot of quality centers will actually complete multiple reviews as standard practice, so more eyes will be assessing the subtleties of your films. And finally, it's essential that your radiologists compare your current films to prior ones, as changes in breast composition or texture should be identified and evaluated thoroughly.

- *The equipment.* Check to make sure that the machine that you will receive your mammogram from is state-of-the-art. Many institutions have a variety of machines, but you will always want the latest technology.
- *The technician.* While the person who takes your images should help you feel as comfortable and calm as possible, it is also important for him or her to be as technically proficient as possible. The more compression of your breast, the better the image quality will be. So if it's not at least slightly uncomfortable, then the technician wasn't securing the most accurate image possible. However, a mammogram should never be painful, except perhaps around the surgery incision site.

Regardless of where you live, even in fairly remote rural areas, you should be able to locate a top-flight radiology facility within a couple hours of your home. Ask your doctor to refer you to a breast clinic with a reputable breast radiology department that conducts a high volume of breast imaging on a daily basis. Then, make it a special day, an annual outing that you deserve, to give yourself the best health care possible. If possible, tie it in to other activities, such as shopping, a special cultural event, or a family gathering.

Blood Level Markers: A Way to Keep Score.

While there is no known blood test to determine if cancer has spread beyond the lymph nodes upon initial diagnosis, there are certain "markers" that your oncologist will look for by drawing blood at each checkup. If elevated, these *may*, or may not, indicate a systemic recurrence. Markers are proteins released by *some*, not all, tumor cells into the blood that may reflect the volume of tumor in the body. These proteins, however, are also released by normal tissues and may rise for nonmalignant reasons such as smoking, viral syndromes, and many others. The two most prevalent tests look for elevated levels of either: (a) CEA, a carcinoembryonic antigen, or (b) CA15-3 (or CA 27-29) to determine if further testing is warranted.

Carrying the Breast Cancer Gene: Do You Really Want to Know? And When?

Since my name is Cohen (clearly Jewish) and my relatives are from Yugoslavia and other parts of Eastern Europe (clearly Ashkenazic Jew), my oncologist first mentioned the concept of genetic testing at our initial consultation: "Oh, by the way, you don't need to do anything right this moment, but when you're through with treatment, we should probably test you for the breast cancer gene. Given your young age at diagnosis, and your family heritage, I'd guess there's a thirty percent chance you carry the gene." As my jaw dropped open in astonishment, my initial reaction was "Please, just don't even go there." I was completely emotionally incapable of even thinking that there would be a way to predict my future experiences with cancer, should there be any. Getting through today was enough.

Apparently Ashkenazic Jewish women have a statistically greater chance of carrying this "breast cancer gene" than others. What this actually *means* is the crux of the debate (see "A Note from the Oncologist," below.) But the more fundamental question is, "What would you do about it if you tested positive?" The answer to that is an extremely personal decision based on a host of complex factors that should be discussed with a geneticist. In deciding whether or not to go through genetic testing, a few issues to wrestle with include:

- *Emotional impact.* Do you want to know if you are predisposed to further "female" cancers in your life (e.g., breast cancer in your healthy breast or ovarian cancer)? Or do you want to live without the potential burden of a positive diagnosis, just leading a full, healthy life, living for every day as it comes? Or would you like the relief that might come with learning of a negative diagnosis (which remember, doesn't mean you won't get cancer). Which is easier for you to digest, knowing or not knowing?

- *Actions to take.* Perhaps most important, what, if any, actions would you take if you learned you carried BRCA1 or BRCA2? Would you consider a preventative mastectomy in the non-cancerous breast? Would you consider an oophorectomy to prevent ovarian cancer? Do you still want children or are you finished with your family? If you would take no action, then why would you want to carry the possible burden of negative news?

- *Family impact.* How might your family dynamics be disrupted? What type of guilt might your parents feel if they were to learn you inherited a faulty gene from them? If you have daughters, what type of guilt might you feel knowing you could have passed this to them? Are your family relationships strong enough to handle this?

- *Financial impact.* Since most testing today is done in utmost confidence by your medical provider, and not even filed with your insurance company, do you have the funds to spend? Is it worth it to possibly sleep easier at night if you're not a carrier? Or would you decide to file with your insurance carrier, knowing that this record could now be made available to a variety of people, including possible employers, other insurance companies, and other places it could cause you discriminatory problems?

- *Timing.* When would you want to do this? Immediately after getting through your treatment? At your five-year survival mark, when you're more certain you'll be around for the long term? Or perhaps when you're done having children, are through menopause, and would be willing to part with your reproductive organs?

A NOTE FROM THE ONCOLOGIST

R̥ BRCA1 AND BRCA2: A Default in the
Genetic Road Map of Life

So what is this "breast cancer gene," and how can it possibly predict the disposition to a breast cancer diagnosis? DNA
is material that resides in each cell in your body and contains
the genetic "blueprint" which determines how your body grows
and develops. Consider it the software that instructs your
body how to live. Of the 200,000 genes a person is born with
(100,000 pairs, with one from each parent), two—BRCA1 and
BRCA2—have been identified to be two of the genes that can
cause breast cancer later in life.

Approximately 5–10 percent of all women diagnosed with
breast cancer have received a defective, or "mutant," BRCA1 or
BRCA2 gene from one of their parents (note then that the
overwhelming majority of all breast cancers are *not* genetically
rooted). Up to 80 percent of the women with BRCA1 will develop breast cancer at some point in their life, and up to 60
percent will develop ovarian cancer. Note that the statistics
vary slightly according to which report you read, but they are
all in this ballpark.

Oncologists and genetic counselors use several criteria to
determine who might be an appropriate "high-risk" candidate,
including breast and/or ovarian patients who: (a) have two or
more first- or second-degree relatives with breast or ovarian
cancer, (b) have one relative with breast or ovarian cancer at
younger than age 45, (c) have breast or ovarian cancer themselves at younger than age 45, or (d) have had more than one
primary tumor.[5] It is a good idea to have the test performed
by a genetic counselor.

5. OncorMed, "Comparison of the 'Statement of the American Society of Clinical
Oncology: Genetic Testing for Cancer Susceptability' to OncorMed's Institutional Review
Board Approved Protocols for BRCA1/BRCA2 and HNPCC Testing," OncorMed, Inc., 205
Perry Parkway, Gaithersburg, MD 20877, 301-208-1888, February 1997.

LONGER-TERM ISSUES: THE AFTERMATH

So, Will My "Normal" Ob-Gyn Visits Ever Be "Normal" Again?

Your so-called "routine" ob-gyn visits might become a bit more complicated after breast cancer treatment. Two factors driving this are: (a) chemotherapy may have thrown your hormone system off-balance for a while, resulting in menopausal-like symptoms, and (b) you may be at slightly higher risk for certain reproductive cancers so you'll need to be watched more closely than the average patient. So, here are a few things to discuss with your gynecologist to make sure you maintain a healthy reproductive system:

- *Pap smears.* While routine pap smears test for cervical cancers, if you were on chemotherapy, your pap smears may indicate abnormal results due to the effect of chemotherapy on the cells of your cervix. Don't be alarmed if your pap smear doesn't return with "normal" results during or shortly after chemotherapy. However, they should return to normal within a year.
- *Menopausal symptoms.* Chemotherapy might cause menopausal-like symptoms. Depending on your age, this might be the initiation of premature permanent menopause, or just symptoms that will disappear with time, as your hormonal system returns to normal. If you have any of the symptoms such as hot flashes or vaginal dryness, talk with your doctor about means to minimize the discomfort. (See Chapter 7, "Managing Physical Side Effects [of Chemotherapy]," for more.) And be patient. It might take a year or more to resume full ovulation and menstruation.
- *Vaginal sonograms.* Since you might be at higher risk for ovarian cancer, discuss the possibility of an annual vaginal sonogram in addition to your routine pelvic exam. Ovarian cancer is generally scarier than breast cancer because it is more difficult to detect at early stages. A sonogram is one such tool that can at least attempt to monitor this. If nothing else, it will provide you with a comfort level that you're taking action for prevention.

- *Annual mammograms.* Regardless of your age, once you're a breast cancer survivor, you should have a mammogram at least annually. Also, any breast lumps, whether detected by self-exam or on mammograms, will be evaluated more aggressively. It would be very rare for your doctor to say to you upon discovery of a lump, "Let's wait a few months to see if it disappears."
- *Monitoring tamoxifen.* If you are taking tamoxifen, your gynecologist will want to watch for uterine cancer, either semiannually or annually. Many gynecologists will monitor you with vaginal ultrasound and may even conduct an endometrial biopsy for any bleeding or nonreassuring sonograms. In an endometrial biopsy, a sample of tissue is removed from the uterine wall and analyzed for any potential cancerous cells.

The Continued Importance of Breast Self-Exams.

The importance of monthly breast self-exams, even as a survivor, can never be overstated. The more familiar you are with the contours and textures of your breasts, and variations during your monthly cycle, the better off you will be. The objective is not to diagnose a condition—that's your doctor's job—but to be aware enough of any changes to bring them to your doctor's attention.

New Considerations for Pregnancy.

If you're like me, you always thought that getting pregnant and bringing a child into the world would be one of life's most special experiences as a woman. Well, it still is, but when you're a cancer survivor, there are some very real factors to consider that quickly bring you back to reality of the stress it places on your body. If you have made it through treatment without experiencing menopause, and if you are young enough that you are still in the family planning phase of your life, there are a few things to evaluate regarding if, when, and how to get pregnant:

- *Estrogen-receptor status of cancer cells.* If your cancer cells were estrogen-receptor positive, it may be riskier for you to get pregnant. With the hormonal surges associated with pregnancy, both estrogen and progesterone, any dormant cancer cells may be awakened to become active.

- *Impact of chemotherapy on ovaries.* At birth, every woman is born with a full complement of eggs in her ovaries to last a lifetime, releasing one or more during menstrual cycle. However, chemotherapy can damage ovaries in a variety of ways. Even if you didn't experience menopause, chemotherapy may kill some eggs completely, or may have chromosomally damaged your remaining eggs, so they may be incapable of fertilization or may cause genetic defects. To some extent, a fertility specialist can determine the quality of your eggs, and whether you have a chance at a successful pregnancy.

- *Length of survival.* While there is a bit of debate, some oncologists recommend that you wait until you're past your five-year survival mark to consider pregnancy due to the impact it may have on your body. However, others are comfortable with pregnancy as soon as two years postcancer.

- *Limited fertility options.* You might be unable to get pregnant the natural way, for a variety of reasons, some of which may have nothing to do with your cancer history. But as a cancer survivor, your options for fertility treatments become restricted, as many fertility programs include significant hormone stimulation, and that is not something your oncologist is going to smile at. So, you may need to think a bit more creatively about how to have children, even though they may not be your genetic children. Egg donor pregnancies are increasing in success rates, and adoption is always an option. You just need to remember the end goal. Do you want to be a healthy parent? Do you need to have your own genetic child? Do you need to experience pregnancy?

If you decide to get pregnant, you should consult with your oncologist, gynecologist, and perhaps even a fertility specialist. You might also contact any of the breast cancer organizations and ask to be referred to women who are willing to talk about choices they have made concerning pregnancy. Not only is this an emotion-laden decision, but there is not much of a fact base to rely on. Although it is an area of increasing focus, to date there has been minimal clinical research that has studied whether pregnancy increases the risk of recurrence in young breast cancer survivors over the long term. So your doctors will not have a definitive recommendation for you. It will be a very personal decision, in which you must balance the

206 — Getting Back to Life

fear of unknown potential risks associated with the hormonal surges of pregnancy with the psychological benefits and joy of sustaining and perpetuating life. Young survivors who have gone on to have children unanimously cite pregnancy as one of the most life-affirming decisions they could have made in their ongoing quest for health.

If You Truly Want to Be a Parent, Adoption Is Always a Wonderful Option.

If you do face obstacles in becoming pregnant after breast cancer, remember adoption as an alternative means to parenthood. Perhaps it was coincidence, or perhaps it was fate, but concurrent with my own breast cancer experience, one of my closest friends was riding the emotional roller coaster of trying to become a parent. After many rounds of infertility treatments, she and her husband turned to adoption, and ended up with a wonderful baby boy. Whenever I see them, she keeps reminding me, "In a strange way, I'm glad I didn't get pregnant, because Jamie was meant to be my son. We couldn't have 'made' a better one ourselves."

So, if parenthood is your end goal, and pregnancy doesn't seem to be the route there, investigate adoption by asking around. Your doctors, social workers, support group members, and other research sources discussed throughout this book should be able to refer you to adoption information and support groups that will help you investigate options. "Resolve" is one such national resource network that you might inquire about.

Finding Replacements for Estrogen-Replacement Therapy.

By now, once you've been through treatment, you've most likely been taken off any estrogen replacement therapy (ERT) you were on to manage menopause. However, that doesn't mean that you must sacrifice the well-known long-term benefits of such drugs, including prevention of heart disease and osteoporosis. While ERT is not monolithically ruled out for you, your gynecologist might want to discuss more individualized alternatives that compartmentalize each of the benefits. For example, you might use calcium and weight-bearing exercise programs to combat osteoporosis, and develop another alternative for mitigating potential heart disease. New medications that promote calcium restoration in bone and do not have the risks of traditional ERT are available and widely used.

You're Not a Hypochondriac—Just a Bit of Posttraumatic Stress Syndrome.

Part of the aftermath of the breast cancer experience is very similar to the posttraumatic stress syndrome often experienced by war survivors. In either case, you become extremely paranoid about repeating a horrible experience. Just as a soldier might jump out of his skin with terror every time he hears a ticking sound behind him, convinced it's a bomb, so might you become somewhat of a hypochondriac. But that's okay. You wouldn't have normal survival instincts if you didn't. Every time you have a pain in your joints or bones, you'll be sure it's cancer, rather than just a simple inflammation or strain. And worse yet, if you ever have an abnormal test result for any medical condition, you'll be convinced you have a recurrence. Calm down. Manage your anxiety by telling yourself it's normal to be panicked. And don't ever think an ache or pain is too small to mention to one of your doctors, especially if it lasts more than a couple weeks.

TRANSITIONING BACK TO "NORMAL"

Take a Vacation. You Deserve It.

When you are ready, both physically and emotionally, go someplace unusual, or do something different that clearly delineates the end of your treatment and your return to daily life. Celebrate normalcy. For a lot of women, that means a vacation. Just going away will be refreshing and make you feel that your life has been given back to you, as most women aren't allowed to travel far from their health care team during treatment. I—along with many other women I spoke with—went to a health spa with a friend, which served a dual purpose for me. First, I felt like it was a final, thorough cleansing of all the treatment toxins from my body, and second, it was the beginning of a disciplined program to regain my former strength and energy. Take a week. Don't feel guilty.

Your Physical Return to Normalcy: A Five o'Clock Shadow and Ten Little Eyelashes.

Everyone will tell you their own theory of how long it will take for your body to return to normal after chemotherapy. The most telling signal is your hair (if you lost most or all of it). Take bets. You might make some money off it. The bets placed on me ranged from "right away" to "six to eight weeks." I was even cautioned by my wig fitter, "Honey, your little hair follicles have been asleep for a long time, and it may take them a while to wake up and get going." Reading between the lines, I interpreted this as "Brace yourself, it could be several months." Relax. You haven't had hair in several months anyway. But believe me, when it decides to reappear, it will make a grand entrance. About six weeks after completing chemotherapy, I awoke one morning to find a five o'clock shadow all over my head! Additionally, you might reverse the countdown of your eyelashes on your lid (I had been down to eight remaining on my left eye, and suddenly I saw ten)! You'll be so excited that you'll want to throw the wigs and the makeup out the window. Don't just yet. You might still scare someone. The lesson? Absolutely nobody can predict how long any one individual's body will take to restore itself.

Regaining Mental Clarity. It Really Wasn't All in Your Head (or Maybe It Was).

Throughout treatment, many women sense a very vague, but very real change in their ability to think clearly, concentrate, and/or focus. And they are often hesitant to discuss these changes with their doctors, who oftentimes will pass them off as mild depression, anxiety, or even a figment of their imagination. It may not have been your imagination, but rather a very real change in the chemistry of your brain. Although it has not been extensively studied to date, many doctors will admit that sometimes the chemicals used in treatment have a very real effect on mental clarity. So if you find yourself with a renewed or greater sense of concentration and clarity, enjoy it. The fog has lifted and you are returning to "normal."

Exercise: Moving It Up on the Priority List.

If you haven't yet heard about the tremendous benefits of exercise for overall health, wellness, and disease prevention, your name is probably Rip Van Winkle and you've been asleep in a cave for the past twenty years. So I'm not going to spend a lot of time persuading you to start or continue a regular exercise program. Rather, I'd hope that your breast cancer experience helps you keep daily exercise and good physical condition a top priority in your life, rather than letting it slip behind ten other competing priorities.

But just in case you need a little additional incentive, the theory behind the benefit of exercise in keeping breast cancer at bay has three important aspects. First, exercise may stimulate the immune system's ability to detect and destroy defective cells such as cancer. Second, exercise may inhibit the production of a tumor-stimulating form of estrogen (C-16), which has been found to form at double the normal rate in women with breast cancer. While there have been several studies looking at various aspects of exercise and cancer, there is not yet one definitive study on the relationship between exercise and breast cancer. However, one of the most extensive study to date is a fourteen-year trial of 26,000 healthy Norwegian women, ages 20–54, who exercised at least four times per week.[6] Even after accounting for diet and other lifestyle factors, these women had half the incidence of breast cancer as the more sedentary control group. And third, it is a tremendous source of stress reduction and anxiety management, as exercise stimulates the production of endorphins, chemicals in your brain that produce a sense of well-being (while also strengthening the immune system). So get moving, stay fit, and stay well.

Regain the Equilibrium in Your Relationships.

There's been an incredible ebb and flow of people in and out of your life over the past several months, but it may be time for some rebalancing to reestablish a steadier state. Perhaps your phone won't be ringing off the hook as often with people "just checking in," but consider that a good thing. No, you may not be the center of attention anymore, but everyone still has you very much at the

6. *MAMM Magazine,* October/November 1997, p. 71.

forefront of their thoughts and prayers. They just feel the immediate crisis has past, and they're confident you can handle your day-to-day needs again. You'll also reach a transition point where you want people around, but more for social reasons rather that just caretaking and support. Start taking the initiative again with those who have been there. Show your family and friends how much you've valued them.

No, You Can't Return to Your Regularly Scheduled Programming.

You will most likely fail at building a fulfilling life if you just try to "get back to normal," to pretend that your cancer experience didn't happen, that it's behind you, and that it didn't change you. Sorry, it's not that easy. Your cancer experience will change you profoundly, in ways that you may not discern for many months to come. Use it as a tremendous learning experience, as an opportunity to evaluate what works and doesn't work in your life and to make some changes. For many women, cancer gives them the courage to walk away from bad relationships. For others, a more rewarding, meaningful career transition is called for. And others just do a bit of reprioritizing, spending more time on their children or less time on the more superfluous relationships in their lives. What's important becomes crystal clear. Resume old passions you may have buried. Remind yourself of the focusing principles, of those core beliefs in your life. Integrate the experience into the rest of your life.

Emotional Impact: An Attitude Adjustment Is in Order.

I found that when I tried to go back to my normal life, I needed a bit of an attitude adjustment to deal with the inherent frustrations and more mundane details of this daily activity we call living. I felt like such a hero, like I had overcome such an inordinate challenge, that I had absolutely no tolerance for the petty or insignificant. I found myself repeatedly in situations where I'd think, "Get over it. There are worse problems in the world, like cancer!" Whether it was a friend ruminating on her relationship woes or the usual office politics or some other shenanigans, I just had no patience. It took me a while to realize that in the context of these individuals' lives, their woes were meaningful and real. I had to get off my soapbox, overcome my holier-than-thou attitude, and regain the empathy and understanding that had made me a valued friend or colleague in the first place. But now I came at things with a lot calmer and wiser perspective.

Fear of Recurrence? Of Course.

Yes, you will have moments of panic. You wouldn't be normal if you didn't. But then, move on and forget about it for the moment. Remind yourself how lucky you were to have caught the cancer early this time. And convince yourself that by the time you should ever have a recurrence, if you do, there will be new treatments, perhaps even a cure, as the advancement in understanding of this disease is moving at lightning speed. Live your life and plot your future. Think about being the elderly, eccentric woman who wears purple and eats pickles in my favorite poem, "Warning" by Jenny Joseph. Decide what color you want to wear. Because you'll hopefully be there someday.

A Mere "How Are You?" Becomes a Very Loaded Question.

For years after breast cancer, particularly with people you haven't seen in a while, the harmless greeting that is at the core of our social interchange, "How are you?," becomes a very loaded question on both sides. How you respond is a delicate judgment call, based on the precise meaning of those three little words. From your inquirer's perspective, most people want everything to be back to normal and want you to tell them you're okay. They really don't plan to hear otherwise. However, occasionally, this question will be a gentle way of letting you know that if you want to talk, they're willing to listen. Evaluate the intonation. A rushed "How-are-you?" is very different from a prolonged, emphatic "How *are* you?" From your perspective, use your response as a signal about how much you want to disclose. A cursory "I'm great, thank you" can indicate exactly that, or that you just don't feel like talking right now, whereas a "I'm coping just fine, thanks" is a bit more revealing that you understand their concern, but there's nothing really new to report right now.

Breast Cancer Is Not Your New Identity. Remember All Those Wonderful Attributes of Who You Were "before BC."

By the time you're through treatment, you may feel as if you've become the poster child/woman for breast cancer. Your primary label has been "the woman who's going through breast cancer" for so long that you wonder if it has permanently superseded "friend," "confidant," "wife," "mother," "daughter," "sister," "neighbor," "professional colleague," _____ (fill in your job title if you have one), or any other role you play in this journey we call life. Don't let breast cancer become your new identity. Breast cancer advocate and educator is a potential new role you might appropriately add to your repertoire (if you find it rewarding). But remember all those wonderful attributes you had before breast cancer. They're all still there. It's just time for a rearrangement of roles and attributes from "before BC" to "BC" and now to "after BC."

Hi Ho, Hi Ho, It's Back to Work I Go . . . Oh No?

The transition back to a full immersion in your workplace is often a bit challenging regardless of whether you took actual physical leave during your treatment or not. Even if you worked throughout to maintain your sense of routine, you may have had a less than full load, and you were probably distracted by the logistics of doctors' appointments and anxieties about your treatments and side effects. You weren't all there mentally. So when it's time to focus on work again, many women have a strange experience. They agree that it feels good to be "back to normal" and regain that sense of accomplishment, worth, value, respect, and even challenge that a workplace provides. Yet, they don't feel like they fit in anymore. Since the cancer experience often clarifies life's priorities and values, you may have moved on, while work remained static. So it may be time for a career transition, to something you've been pondering for a while, to something that you haven't had the courage, focus, or tenacity to pursue until now. If work doesn't seem like what it used to be, remember, your world has changed.

If you do decide to make a move, don't act too impulsively or abruptly. Do your homework and take your time, for two reasons.

First, for a couple years, you will still be on a roller coaster of emotions, so you don't want to do anything you might regret later. And second, scrutinize your health insurance plans and conditions for coverage should you change employers.

Long-Term Plans, and Celebrating 40?

Another signal of the return to normalcy is the restored ability to focus on the future, to think about the longer term without sheer terror. You also develop a different perspective on the long term. For example, I used to dread my fortieth birthday, which seemed to be creeping up all too quickly, as years of my life seemed to be whizzing by. Like most people, I planned to run away to a desert island with a few friends and forget about it. However, since my fortieth will now be the same as my five-year survival mark, it will be the biggest celebration I've ever hosted. And I'll savor every year until I get there. Isn't it interesting how your life perspective changes? Don't worry about the long term. But do celebrate it when you get there.

You Know You've Arrived When . . . The Transition from "Patient" to "Survivor."

The defining moment when you know, consciously or not, that you've conquered your breast cancer and completed this phase of your life journey is when you refer to yourself as a survivor rather than a patient. It might just slip out of your mouth in conversation. Or a light bulb might go off in your head, triggered by a defining event such as your first visit back to your oncologist for a follow-up visit. Or someone else may refer to you as a survivor in the context of asking your assistance in guiding another woman who has been newly diagnosed. Utilize the opportunity not only to help someone, but also as proof to yourself of the distance you've come since you were "there." Give yourself perspective. Regardless of how the moment becomes defined, consider it a milestone. Just like the defining moment of your initial diagnosis is indelibly embedded as part of your heritage, mark the move to survivor as well.

Chapter 9
Maintaining a Healthy Lifestyle: The Long-Term Outlook

Once you've been through cancer, how you regard your body and nourish it takes on a whole new perspective. Never again will you take your health for granted. And never again will you be able to feel invincible, to think that you can abuse your body—be it from stress, lack of sleep, inactivity, poor nutrition, or smoking or drinking—which are now completely off your list of vices! Your body becomes a holy temple, which you now need to revere and worship. You need to maintain both the physical and the emotional strength to handle whatever challenges life may deal you. So, this very last chapter offers some guidance on:

- *Nutrition,* or looking at food in an entirely different way, as essential fuel for your body.
- Navigating the maze of *Alternative Medicine* and how to find approaches and modalities that work for you in optimizing your health over the long term.

NUTRITION: LOOKING AT FOOD IN AN ENTIRELY DIFFERENT WAY

It seems that every day, there is a new study released to the media making sweeping claims that some food, vitamin, herb, or mineral is either miraculously good or disastrously dangerous for your health. It is all so confusing and difficult to track that you are beginning to think that it might be easiest if the FDA just came out and proclaimed, "Warning: Eating May Be Hazardous to Your Health!" Relax. There really are some fairly simple, straightforward guidelines about how to build a diet strong in the basic nutrients, vitamins, minerals, and other compounds that contribute to overall good health. Looking out for your total health will ensure that at the very least, you're getting enough of the "anticancer elements"—those antioxidants and other compounds—that may work to prevent abnormal cells from becoming cancerous cells and forming tumors. There are also a few simple tricks to ensure that whatever you're putting in your body is as pure as possible. This section will help you develop your own list of simple nutritional guidelines.

Nutrition: An Essential Weapon in Your Anticancer Arsenal.

For any woman wanting to maintain optimum health, which includes disease prevention in addition to wellness, there are a few basic principles of good nutrition:

- *Control calories to control weight.* You'll want to maintain a calorie intake level sufficient for good nutrition, but that keeps you from being overweight. Some research studies show a correlation between obesity and breast cancer, as fat can encourage estrogen production, which can trigger breast cancer cell growth. Others, however, remain inconsistent. Nevertheless, limiting your fat intake may help your cancer cause, and will definitely help your weight control cause. So start counting those calories and fat grams!
- *Maintain a 60–20–20 balance of your macronutrients (carbohydrate, protein, and fat).* Macronutrients are among the substances that are essential to support life. They are required in fairly significant amounts on a regular basis, as they are the substances that undergo chemical transformation to sustain and fuel our bodies. Breast cancer survivors should maintain a balance among the three main macronutrients of:
    - *60 percent carbohydrates,* which provide energy for our bod-

ies to function, but excess becomes stored as fat—rich sources include whole grain pastas and breads; individual grains such as rice, barley, and quinoa; or fruits and vegetables.

- *20 percent protein,* which is essential to maintaining a healthy immune system, and creating and repairing vital cells in the body. Rich sources are "complete proteins" such as fish, poultry, and eggs, but also can be found in grains, nuts, seeds, beans, and other legumes such as lentils.

- *No more than 20 percent fat,* which is sufficient to help the body absorb nutrients and perform other functions. Excess should be avoided—try to restrict your fats to monounsaturated fats such as canola or olive oils, and substitute red meat with fish, as it contains certain "essential fatty acids" that contribute to health.

- *Eat 5–9 servings of fruits and vegetables daily.* While fruits and veggies supply some of the macronutrients discussed above, they also supply a wealth of micronutrients, those vitamins and minerals that act as the "spark plugs" that transform macronutrients into energy for your body. Certain vitamins, particularly A, C, and E, are good antioxidants, those substances that protect the body's cells from damage (see "A Note from the Oncologist").

- *Eat at least 25 grams of fiber daily.* Fiber is good for your digestive system, ensuring that important nutrients get absorbed by your body, as well as providing a range of general health benefits. Specific to breast cancer, the theory is that fiber binds to excess estrogen in the intestinal tract, which can then be eliminated from the body.[7] Your fruits and vegetables will help meet your daily fiber requirements.

- *Ensure sufficient calcium intake.* All women need calcium to optimize bone health and reduce the risk of osteoporosis. For premenopausal women, the recommended daily amount is 1,000 mg, taken with 200 IU of vitamin D to maximize absorption. Postmenopausal women require higher levels: 1,500 mg calcium with 400 IU vitamin D. Try to get your requirements met through calcium-intensive foods like low-fat yogurt, milk, and cheese, only supplementing where you fall short.

7. *The Breast Cancer Survival Manual,* p 116.

A NOTE FROM THE ONCOLOGIST

R̥ **Antioxidants: Part of Your Body's Defense Mechanisms**

It seems that you can't get through a conversation on cancer prevention without being lectured on the benefits of antioxidants. So what are they, and now that you actually have cancer, what are they doing for you? Antioxidants behave like scavengers of "free radicals," neutralizing them before they can do any damage to a cell's components. Free radicals are by-products of the normal process of metabolism—yes, everybody has them—which are "unstable" because they are missing an electron (remember those negatively charged particles from science class). These unstable compounds undergo an "oxidation" process in which they take and transfer electrons, leaving behind a new free radical. This process can cause enormous damage to your body's cells, and will continue unless an "antioxidant" halts the process. While the body has its own defenses against the oxidation process, foods rich in vitamins A, C, and E contribute greatly to the cause. However, keep in mind that under certain conditions or taken to the extreme, any antioxidant can have negative effects. So, as with your general diet, keep it in balance, and don't overdo it! And don't take anything *during* chemotherapy or radiation without checking with your doctor.

As Always, Variety Is the Spice of Life.

As with many aspects of life, variety is the key to success. If you eat a wide variety of proteins and carbohydrates, with an emphasis on fruits and vegetables, you will be eating a well-balanced diet. Variety also provides another benefit. It will ensure that you are getting the micronutrients—those essential vitamins and minerals—that are believed to have "anticancer" properties as well as contribute to overall good health. A few foods rich in these compounds that you might want to incorporate into your diet include garlic, onions, and mushrooms.

Phytochemicals: A Collection of Confusing Terms . . . with Health Benefits.[8]

You may receive advice from all sorts of people who want to provide you with that "miracle diet" that will prevent your cancer from recurring. In addition to your head spinning from too many well-intentioned people with too much advice, you may also be confused by very complex-sounding ingredients in food that you are supposed to put in your body. In a nutshell, most of these "disease-preventing" substances can be grouped under a category called "phytochemicals." Simply put, they are "plant chemicals," or those compounds found in very small amounts that interact with the basic nutrients discussed above in very complex but powerful ways to prevent disease and boost overall health.

Although the medical community is just beginning to study the specific role of these substances in health, a heavily plant-based diet (e.g., fruits, veggies) has been advocated for many years. Although we don't know exactly how everything works, scientists are beginning to believe that phytochemicals may fight cancer in a variety of ways, from suppressing cells exposed to carcinogenic substances from turning cancerous, to preventing the formation of new blood vessels capable of carrying fuel to a growing tumor, to boosting the overall immune system.

A few types of phytochemicals that are considered "anticancer" wonders are listed below. However, instead of being paralyzed by trying to remember which phytochemicals are contained in which foods, just ignore the specific names, and make sure you get an abundant, varied supply of these foods in your diet:

- *Common phytochemicals:* carotenoids, coumarins, flavonoids, indoles, lignans, isoflavones (including genistein and daidzen), organosulfurs, and phytosterols.
- *Phytochemical-rich foods:* red, green, yellow, and orange vegetables, including carrots, sweet potatoes, and tomatoes; cruciferous vegetables such as broccoli, cabbage, and kale; dark leafy greens, such as spinach or romaine lettuce; fruits, including citrus fruits and berries; flaxseeds; whole grains and legumes; garlic; onions; leeks; soybeans and soybean products such as tofu and soy milk; and green tea and other herbal teas.

8. *PowerFoods,* Stephanie Beling, M.D., HarperCollins Publishers, Inc., 1997, pp. 8–27.

Broccoli (Almost) Every Day Keeps the Doctor Away.

In late 1998, a stalk of broccoli appeared on the cover of *Newsweek* magazine, as part of a cancer prevention article. If not touted as the miracle cure for cancer, it came only a small step short. Packed with phytochemicals, the entire cruciferous family of vegetables offers some of the best possible nutritional defense against breast cancer. The theory is that one of the chemical compounds in cruciferous vegetables changes the way estrogen is metabolized.[9] I try to get at least one serving daily of either broccoli, kale, leeks, Brussels sprouts, cauliflower, collard greens, or cabbage. No, not all are my favorites, but I consider them medicine rather than food, which makes them go down a bit easier.

Bright Orange and Dark Green: A Color Combination You'll Grow Quite Fond Of.

Another group of foods packed with "anticancer" vitamins and phytochemicals include the red, orange, and yellow vegetables; the dark leafy greens; and a few fruits as well. By attempting to make my meals as colorful as possible, I guarantee inclusion of vitamins A, C, and E, as well as beta-carotene, all important antioxidants. Think about including apricots, peaches, melons, squashes, sweet potatoes, yams, carrots, and pumpkin in your orange grouping, and spinach and the dark lettuces in your green grouping.

Use Flaxseed When You Don't Have Time for Salmon.

In addition to being a good source of fiber, flaxseed is being studied for a whole host of health benefits, from heart disease to cancer prevention. Flaxseed contains high concentrations of omega-3 fatty acids, a type of essential fatty acid, the same element contained in fish, that has been touted as a strong anticancer food. If possible, get at least a few servings of fish such as salmon, mackerel, and swordfish each week. As a supplement, you can also sprinkle flaxseeds onto just about anything—salads, cereals, yogurt, vegetables, pastas. They're tasteless. Just make sure to grind them up first, to release the oils and maximize the health benefits. You can also take flaxseed oil in capsule or liquid form.

9. *The Breast Cancer Survival Manual*, p. 118.

Tofu, Tempeh, or Miso . . . As Long As You Get Your Soy.

You might have heard by now that Asian women have the lowest incidence of breast cancer in the world, and researches have pointed to their diets as the probable reason. Not only is the Asian diet low in fat and plentiful in vegetables and fish (for those omega-3 fatty acids), but it also is rich in soy. Soy products contain phyto-estrogens (plant estrogens), particularly the phytochemicals genistein and diadzein. These phytochemicals may help reduce breast cancer risk by binding to estrogen receptor sites on cells and replacing stronger estrogens.

Since it can be found in many forms, soy can easily be incorporated into your daily food intake as part of an overall well-balanced diet. (Don't go soy crazy!) Use it in recipes for delicious healthful meals: soy flour, soy milk, soy protein powder (which is mixed into beverages), soybeans, soy nuts for snacks, tofu (soybean curd), tempeh (fermented soybeans and grains), and miso (fermented soybean paste). Or alternatively, if you want ready-to-go soy, search your local grocery store for soy burgers, soy bacon, and soy cheese among other items. However, look carefully at the ingredients to avoid "soy protein concentrate," as the isoflavones have been removed during processing. Stick to foods with "isolated soy protein," or "textured soy protein." And finally, opt for "low-fat" versions if you're concerned about your fat intake. For everything you ever wanted to know about soy, try one of the many soy cookbooks on the market.

Green Tea: Another Ancient Asian Remedy.

Here's a quick and easy anticancer health tip: If you've only thought of green tea as something that comes in those minicups at Chinese restaurants, think again. The ancient Chinese were smart about making green tea a staple of their diet. It's a wonderful source of antioxidants, and generally works to keep the immune system strong. Additionally, if you've given up coffee (more on that shortly), it's a nice replacement, and it does contain some caffeine. And furthermore, it's made its way from the back shelves of health food stores to front and center on the menus at many restaurants and coffeehouses.

A Personal Checklist: Have I Had My Anticancer Foods Today?

Since my lifestyle tends to be chaotic and I don't always have time to prepare and sit down to a meal, I have my own personal checklist of six strong anticancer foods I've chosen—high in antioxidants and compounds that keep the immune system strong. If I can get at least three of the six almost every day, I feel like I'm doing quite well in my personal war. Develop your own list based on foods you like and how easy they are for you to obtain. My list includes:

- *Soy milk*—easily replaces regular milk with cereal in the morning, a strong start to the day (remember to use the low-fat version).
- *Green tea*—easy to sip on throughout the day, either hot or iced, and easy to carry with you.
- *Carrots or dried apricots*—both easy to keep in the house and carry with you as a snack.
- *Flaxseeds*—also easy to keep in the house or carry with you to sprinkle on vegetables, salads, pastas, cereals. Keep a small container in your desk to use at lunch.
- *Broccoli or cabbage*—both easy to order in restaurants as a hot side vegetable or as part of a salad.
- *Sweet potato or melon* (depending on the season)—the least portable of my group, but both delicious. They are easy to keep in your house, and can be prepared in less than five minutes.

Keep Foods Pure for Maximum Nutritional Benefit and Minimal Added Chemicals.

Purity is generally a good thing, and especially so when it comes to healthy eating. If you can eat foods that are as close to their purest, original state as possible, you'll reap the maximum nutritional benefit. You'll also avoid ingesting many types of chemicals, from artificial sweeteners to preservatives. Although the scientific community is still debating the potential dangers of food additives, my own personal view is simply that my body doesn't need any additional chemicals, especially after treatment. And besides, who knows what they might do to you? A few broad guidelines to follow:

- *Use organic produce, if feasible.* If you can get organic fruits and vegetables where you live easily and economically, great. (However, note that there is no regulation of claims they are to be organic and pesticide-free.) Otherwise, to get rid of the pesticides and other chemicals used in growing them, try using a produce cleaner, which usually comes in spray form, and is available at most health food stores. One brand I like is Healthy Harvest® Fruit & Vegetable Rinse (call 203-245-2033 to locate it). You simply spray your produce, rinse it off, and presto, no more chemicals. An alternative to the spray is to use a small dab of mild, diluted dishwashing liquid, or just run plenty of water over produce to loosen and remove any residue.

- *Eat organic chicken.* Most chicken today is raised commercially, and injected with estrogen, hormones, and antibiotics to make those little chickens plump and meaty for your eating pleasure. Since the last thing any breast cancer patient needs is more estrogen, try to eat organic chicken if possible. I like the Bell & Evans brand, as it tastes wonderful and is widely available at most supermarkets or butchers.

- *Drink 100% natural juices.* Most commercial fruit juices are deceivingly caloric and artificial. But since juice is a quick, easy way to meet your daily fruit requirements, you may want to find juices packed with the most nutrients. Try to stick to apple cider, orange, grapefruit, or pineapple juice, which can easily be obtained as 100% juice. Be careful of so-called juice drinks, as they often contain minimal juice content (10–25%) and are packed with preservatives and artificial sweeteners and flavors.

- *Avoid chemical food substitutes and highly processed foods.* While the media hype around fat and sugar substitutes today promises svelte, thin bodies without giving up junk foods like cookies, chips and sodas, I'm more leery. Who knows what diseases these chemicals will be proven to cause fifty years from now? I've tried to eliminate them from my diet. If I'm going to have cookies, I'd rather have one delicious one, with all-natural ingredients and full fat content, rather than three that claim no-fat, with mediocre flavor. Remember, there's no such thing as a free lunch, so focus on wholesome, natural foods.

Taking Vitamins or Other Supplements: Streamline for Simplicity.

Even with the most healthful of eating patterns, it's often difficult to get the sufficient daily dose of all the antioxidants required given the hectic nature of most people's schedules today. So, you might consider adding a simple multivitamin (low-dose, no high-antioxidant versions, please) to your daily routine. I originally shuddered at the thought of a vitamin program, which for me conjured up images of popping pills ten times a day, swallowing handfuls at a time, and confusing myself over which ones were supposed to be doing what. I had neither the time nor the stomach for that. So, I've simply added a multivitamin before I go to bed at night. Two pills—one multivitamin and one calcium (something all women should take to prevent osteoporosis as they age)—and I'm done.

But in the End, Remember, There's No Substitute for the Real Thing.

If you are considering a more elaborate program of nutritional supplements, consult with both your oncologist and a nutritionist. While deficiencies can cause problems, so can excesses. Just because garlic is a good antioxidant doesn't mean more garlic pills are better. Too much can actually cause toxicity of the liver. Get the proper supervision from a trained professional. Furthermore, and more important, there is a fundamental difference between nutrition from a well-balanced diet and remedial attempts in pill form. In the complex composition of foods, key nutrients interact synergistically to affect absorption rates into the body, and other delicate balances that Mother Nature has perfected. Don't rely on supplements at the expense of your diet. They haven't been approved by Mother Nature.

No Caffeine? Is There a Boycott of Starbucks?

Caffeine can exacerbate breast tenderness and any type of fibrocystic changes (change in the texture of your breast). It can also exacerbate menopausal symptoms like hot flashes, which you might be experiencing either on a temporary or permanent basis. If you suffer from either condition, consider reducing or eliminating your caffeine intake. Okay, so if you're one of those people who can't find their way to the bathroom in the morning without your cup of coffee—or two or three—an occasional cup won't destroy you.

I Really Need a Drink! No, You Don't—Not Anymore.

Even if you've never been a big drinker, given all the trauma and stress of the breast cancer experience, you might find yourself thinking, "I could really use a drink"—even a glass of wine to put you to sleep—more frequently than you used to. Sorry, it's time to temper yourself. (If you went through chemo, you were already on the wagon by your doctor's directive during treatment, so why not just continue?)

Although the specific mechanism is unknown, there's increasing evidence that alcohol consumption increases breast cancer risk. Given this mounting evidence, women who choose to drink are advised to have no more than four servings of alcohol per week. So what about those of us who might not drink daily, but are the occasional weekend social drinker? My oncologist articulated it very simply and emphatically, "The more you drink, the higher the risk!" So, very simply, I don't. Okay, I admit, I do like to enjoy my life. So on special occasions—a wedding, a family birthday, my survival anniversary—I might toast with a glass of wine or champagne, but that's about it.

ALTERNATIVE MEDICINE: IT REALLY CAN HELP

Alternative medicine, holistic medicine, integrative medicine, complementary medicine . . . Confused? So am I! And we haven't even started to discuss specific treatments with hieroglyphic-sounding names like ayurvedic, reiki, shiatsu, or t'ai chi. Once you open the door to alternative medicine, even just a crack to take a peek and perhaps test these unfamiliar waters, you'll feel like a torrent of jargon, philosophies, treatments, and experts has overwhelmed you. You'll be flooded not only with promises of symptom relief, but a return to health and prevention of future disease as well. Can it really be this good? Used appropriately, there must be a reason that many of these medical systems have endured since the genesis of many Eastern religions. However, you may not be sure where to begin, let alone identify the appropriate credentialed professional whom you trust. This section will give a brief definition of alternative medicine and offer perspective on evaluating treatments, as well as some guidance on where to look to determine what might be right for you.

Alternative, Holistic, Integrative, or Complementary Medicine? . . . Just Variations on the East-West Theme.

Physicians, doctors, pharmaceutical drugs, hospitals. These are widely used, well-understood terms that define the traditional Western approach, or "conventional medicine." However, the first point of confusion in venturing into alternative medicine seems to be even what to call it! You may hear any of the following terms used—alternative, holistic, integrative, or complementary—when in reality they are simply variations on the same theme. They differ primarily in how they approach the balance between Eastern and Western medicine. Alternative medicine, for example, strives to avoid conventional Western medical approaches such as surgery or drugs, instead calling on the body's own unique healing powers as an "alternative" way to treat illness and disease. On the other hand, complementary or integrative medicine starts with conventional Western medicine as its foundation, but also seeks out alternative or "complementary" approaches that simultaneously contribute to healing and wellness—essentially a double dosage that can do no harm. You'll hear all sorts of terms, but you just need to decide where you want to start as your foundation approach.

If you do decide to learn the jargon now, you're at the leading edge of a trend. More and more medical schools are adding courses and even entire specialties in non-Western medicine in response to the trend toward more patient-centered care. In this rapidly evolving world of health care, more patients are demanding involvement in their treatment decisions, not just relying on the recommendation of their doctor alone. And one of the key tenets of all types of alternative medicine is extensive patient involvement and commitment.

Eastern versus Western Medicine Doesn't Mean You Need a Compass to Navigate the Basic Principles.

Most of us are most familiar with conventional Western medicine, which is fundamentally based on an "external" approach to addressing disease and bodily malfunctions. In other words, "interventions" such as surgery or drugs are introduced to the body to "fix" the problem or eliminate symptoms. Think of Western medicine as analogous to bringing a broken car to an auto mechanic who will fix the problem with new parts or adjustments but not consider the efficiency of the whole car. Alternatively, Eastern medicine is based on an "internal" approach. Introducing natural substances into the body theoretically "triggers" the body's internal ability to remedy "imbalances" that cause disease, and over the longer term elevates the overall health of the whole person. This is analogous to preventing breakdowns by getting regular tune-ups and making minor adjustments so the car stays in strong working order.

If an "internal" approach to healing is what generically defines Eastern medicine, then there are a few basic principles or tenets common to the many types of alternative medicine.[10]

- *The human body has natural healing powers.* The alternative medical professional believes their role is simply to stimulate those "internal" mechanisms that enable healing.
- *Treatment is patient-centered.* In addition to a medical professional's expertise regarding diagnosis and proposed treatment, an alternative medical professional believes the patient's feelings, beliefs, and opinions are an essential part of determining the most appropriate treatment.
- *Start with the least harmful approach.* Alternative medical professionals believe in beginning with the least invasive and least harmful techniques first, and based on the body's response, moving to more invasive approaches, such as surgery or drugs with potential side effects.
- *Results take longer.* Advocates believe that nature must "take its course" for true healing to occur, which often takes longer than approaches which simply mask symptoms.

10. *Five Steps to Selecting the Best Alternative Medicine: A Guide to Complementary and Integrative Health Care*, Mary and Michael Morton, New World Library, 1996, pp. 11–18.

- *Use natural and whole substances.* Many alternative treatments involve all natural and "whole" substances such as herbs, nutritional supplements, and whole foods under the theory that natural products strengthen the healing process. They also theoretically produce fewer side effects than processed foods or even pharmaceutical drugs, which often are natural substances that are synthesized or chemically treated to be more potent or work faster.

- *Health is more than the absence of illness.* While conventional medicine views health as the absence of disease, alternative practitioners hold health to a higher standard. Many alternative approaches incorporate a concept of a "life force" or "vital energy" that contributes to a person's overall wellness, and affects not only physical, but emotional and mental health as well.

In dealing with a crisis or serious situations such as cancer, the most logical approach is to utilize alternative approaches to supplement conventional efforts, in an attempt to improve the body's overall state of health. I sure wouldn't refuse surgery or chemotherapy because I believed that some tree root or other herb was going to make my cancer disappear! I'd rather take the best of what I can get from where I can get it.

Systems, Modalities, Treatments? A Basic Road Map to Get You to the Appropriate Alternative Medicine Destination for You.

If you are overwhelmed by the plethora of choices of alternative medicine, it might help to take a step back and evaluate a basic framework for how all these seemingly discrete "treatments" fit together to contribute to your health and healing.[11] With examples depicted in the chart below, *systems*, *modalities*, and *treatments* interrelate as follows:

- *Systems.* A system is defined by a core philosophy from which all diagnoses are made, based on a definition of health, an un-

11. *Five Steps to Selecting the Best Alternative Medicine*, p. 127.

derstanding of illness and cures, and an underlying attitude about the meaning of life, among other things. The eight major systems in the world combine modalities and treatments to optimize health.

- *Modalities.* Modalities are seven different approaches used within a system. For example, Traditional Chinese Medicine may incorporate specific treatments from the modalities of diet and nutrition, herbology, and mind/body. Alternatively, conventional Western medicine draws on modalities such as surgery, pharmaceutical drugs, and rehabilitation.
- *Treatments.* Treatments are the specific actions or "tools" the practitioner uses to induce changes in the body that stimulate health and healing.

A ROAD MAP FOR ALTERNATIVE MEDICINE	
Systems	
• Ayurvedic Medicine	• Homeopathy
• Chiropractic	• Naturopathic Medicine
• Environmental Medicine	• Osteopathic Medicine
• Native American Medicine	• Traditional Chinese Medicine
Modalities	
• Bioelectricmagnetic Applications	• Mind/Body Interventions
• Diet and Nutrition	• Pharmacological and Biological Modalities
• Energy Medicine	• Manual Healing
• Herbology/Phytotherapy	
Treatments	
• Acupuncture	• Macrobiotic
• Acupressure Massage	• Nutritional Supplements
• Color/Light Therapy	• Reflexology
• Herbal Treatments	• Shiatsu
• Imagery and Visualization	• T'ai Chi
• Meditation and Relaxation	• Yoga

The Simplest Analogy? A Three-Legged Stool.

If you're still confused by systems, modalities and treatments, think of being able to compare the various approaches to alternative medicine to a three-legged stool, where each leg contributes to the strength of the entire piece. While they all have certain mind/body aspects and there is much overlap, you can think of one leg entailing primarily "physical" activities such as massage, chiropractic, or t'ai chi. A second leg incorporates primarily "spiritual" activities such as meditation, visualization, even prayer. And the third leg simply addresses what you ingest into your body in a deliberate manner, such as nutrition or herb programs.

Why Bother? Optimizing Quality of Life on Two Fronts.

Whether you're considering alternative medicine during or after your treatment phase, you might be feeling a bit overwhelmed and exhausted by doctors. You just can't fathom the thought of dealing with one more doctor, and scheduling one more set of appointments, so you think "Why bother?" Well, if you're concerned about that "overall" level of health we just discussed, and not just the cancer focus, there is a compelling reason to "bother" on two fronts. First, alternative medicine can help maintain your quality of life during the treatment phase by mitigating some of the side effects of chemotherapy (but please make sure you first discuss this with your oncologist). For example, acupuncture has been shown to reduce chemo-induced nausea, and certain herbs are known to mitigate menopausal symptoms related to some drugs such as hot flashes.

And second, after you are through all your treatments, and are officially "discharged" by your oncologist—other than follow-up checkups—and told to return to your "normal" life, alternative medicine can help in two ways. For your physical health, it can perhaps help boost or strengthen your immune system to fight any lingering cancer cells and prevent future occurrences. And equally important, at least for me, it can greatly benefit your mental health. Instead of just being cast back into the world by my oncologists and "waiting" to learn if I'm still healthy fifty years from now, or wondering, "Now what? Am I cured?," I used alternative medicine to empower myself, to help me feel that I had regained control over my body and was doing everything I could to ensure my long-term health.

A Caveat about Herbs: The Fine Line between Plants and Drugs.

Various herbs, and even nutritional supplements, often become trendy and are touted in popular health food stores as nontoxic and nonthreatening to overall health. However, in the case of cancer, you're opening a Pandora's box unless you have the guidance of a trained expert at your side. The more we know about herbs, the more we know that they can have an impact on a variety of cancers in a variety of ways. Something that might be beneficial for another type of cancer may, in fact, be dangerous for breast cancer. Vitamin C is one example where the jury is still out. Furthermore, very different combinations of herbs may be utilized for a specific disease state and type, and even affected by whether you are considering preventative or treatment usage. And finally, since herbs are essentially unregulated—unlike pharmaceuticals—the quality (e.g., potency, purity) varies tremendously. Just as the quality of wine or coffee will vary depending on the origins of the grapes or coffee beans, the cultivation process, and the climate, so, too, will the quality of herbs vary. And remember, the only difference between an herb and many pharmaceutical drugs is that the herbs are in their pure state, but the drugs have been chemically extracted from the original plant, concentrated, and treated. So that's one more reason to find a credentialed expert to guide you through the maze of alternative medicine, and not venture too far on your own.

Write Your Own Song Sheet. But Don't Try to Play the Entire Symphony.

Once you're in the world of alternative medicine, you might become addicted. That is, you might feel compelled to try a bit of everything. Resist the temptation. Pick one or two modalities or types of treatments that work for you, stick with them, and learn to do them well. Imagine the world of alternative medicine as a symphony. It would take many, many years to become proficient at enough different musical instruments so that you could play the entire symphony. And a brief overview course of each instrument wouldn't help you perfect it. So don't. Instead, pick a treatment that complements your personality and natural skill set and work at perfecting it. For example, if you are a dancer, an athlete, or a more physical type of person, you might find yourself drawn to more physical modalities such as yoga or t'ai chi. Alternatively, if you are a more sedentary person, or momentarily feeling too ill to be more active, you might gravitate toward more sedentary modalities like imagery and visualization. Know what works for you on all fronts and make it a lifetime habit.

Finding a Credentialed Expert and Making the Choice. Use Your Health Care Team . . .

Finding an alternative medicine specialist to treat you offers some challenges beyond those faced in assembling your core health care team because more of the burden is on you. First, it's up to you to choose what approaches you might be interested in—mind/body, nutritional, herbs—rather than having the doctor tell you what the protocol dictates. Second, since this world is much less regulated than more traditional fields, the quality of practitioners can vary dramatically. So in choosing your alternative medicine practitioners, not only should you adhere to the original criteria by which you chose your doctors, but you might consider a few other factors as well:

- *Find an M.D. with cancer-specific experience.* If you go to someone who has a background in dealing with the complexities of cancer, and who can integrate alternative therapies with your conventional treatments, you will be much better off. You also won't feel like you are being pulled in opposite directions by different doctors. To identify the best candidates for you, talk to members of your existing health care team, or contact the alternative medicine department of a nearby university medical school.
- *Consider the range of treatments available.* Ideally, you want options to be treated with as many modalities as your doctor thinks appropriate for you, so you want to choose a practitioner who may be trained in multiple areas, or have associ-

ates with a variety of expertise. For example, you may be looking for a Chinese herbalist, but someone who might also be
able to provide or refer you to resources for acupuncture or
mind/body work.

- *Evaluate the attitude toward conventional treatment.* If you
choose an M.D. from the start, this shouldn't really be an issue,
but you want to ensure that your practitioner has an optimistic, cooperative attitude toward conventional medicine.
The last thing you need right now is a dogmatic rebel who believes that the pharmaceutical companies are corrupting traditional doctors. Avoid these types, and find someone who will
cooperate with the rest of your health care team.

- *Test the chemistry.* With alternative medicine, the doctor-
patient relationship is perhaps even more intense than with
traditional medicine, since so much of the treatment is based
on patient feedback (rather than choosing a conventional protocol and abiding by it). Ask for an initial consultation with
any health professional you are considering and make sure the
chemistry is right. Do you want him or her to be your partner
for the foreseeable future?

- *Consider insurance implications.* Be sure to consider the financial and insurance implications of the alternative modalities you are studying. Unfortunately, most are not covered by
insurance plans today, although that is starting to change for
the better. Costs for alternative medicine will vary greatly from
zero for visualization or meditation (once you've learned the
basics) to minor costs associated with monthly supplies of vitamin or herb supplements, to significant costs for bodywork
sessions that might be several times per week.

. . . And Update Your Conventional Medical Team on Your Choices. You May Even Bring Them Some New Insight.

One of the reasons that you probably chose the health care team
you did, particularly your oncologist, was that he or she was interested in your overall well-being. Therefore, he or she will hopefully
be supportive if you decide to investigate complementary therapies.
However, since you are the only one who has the total picture, who

knows every piece of the puzzle you are trying to pull together to heal yourself, please be sure to have a candid discussion with your doctors before you begin any program. They should alert you to any concerns about interference with traditional treatments, and therapies that they might want you to avoid during treatment. However, they should be interested to learn what you are finding helpful. As they hear more and more about complementary techniques their patients believe are effective, it may encourage them to integrate complementary medicine into their traditional practices. You might just bring your doctor some new insight that he or she hadn't even been aware of!

Guides Through the Maze of Alternative Medicine

While I've barely just begun to scratch the surface of the topic of alternative medicine, here are a few references that may provide a more comprehensive overview and frameworks for understanding the wide range of medical systems, philosophies, and programs (for a host of illnesses, not just cancer-related):

Books

• *Five Steps to Selecting the Best Alternative Medicine: A Guide to Complementary and Integrative Health Care,* by Mary and Michael Morton

Cowritten by a couple with two perspectives—his as an alternative doctor, and hers as a patient cured of the chronic spinal condition of scoliosis—this book is a bit alarmist against conventional medicine, which they claim can cause "harm." Despite the tone, it does offer a very easy-to-understand discussion of categories of alternative medicine, how it differs from conventional medicine, a process for identifying appropriate professionals, and an extensive list of organizations and associations to contact for learning more.

• *The Alternative Medicine Handbook: The Complete Reference Guide to Alternative and Complementary Therapies,* by Barrie R. Cassileth, Ph.D.

Since the author was both a founding member of the Office of Alternative Medicine at NIH (see below) and a member of the complementary and alternative medicine committee of the American Cancer Society, she has a great perspective from which to offer a broad-based overview of the landscape of nontraditional treatments. As its title suggests, it's a high-level reference guide with a no-nonsense practical overview that offers a few pages on more than fifty modalities. For each treatment, the following questions are answered: What is it? What do practitioners say it does? What are the beliefs upon which it's based? What's the research evidence to date? What can it do for you? Also included is information on where to get it.

• *Choices in Healing: Integrating the Best of Conventional and Complementary Approaches to Cancer,*
by Michael Lerner, Ph.D.

Probably the closest to a clinical book for the layperson on alternative medicine you'll find, but also extremely informative, comprehensive, and thorough. For those of you who want the entire picture—from background on the historical body of research associated with various "unconventional" cancer treatments to building the case for further research in specific areas—this book is for you. While Lerner clearly argues the need for extensive research in complementary modalities, he also presents the existing debate in a very balanced manner. He is currently President of Commonweal, a health and environmental research institute which he founded in 1976 based on his interests in mind/body health, particularly with regard to cancer.

Organizations

• *National Center for Complementary and Alternative Medicine (NCCAM)*

> NCCAM
> National Institutes of Health (NIH)
> P.O. Box 7923
> Gaithersburg, MD 20898-7923
> Phone: 888-644-6226 (toll-free)
> Web site: www.nccam.nih.gov

As part of the NIH, NCCAM conducts and supports research and training and disseminates information on complementary and alternative medicine to practitioners and the public. It funds thirteen distinct research centers that are looking at various applications of alternative medicine, including the "Center for Alternative Medicine Research in Cancer" at the University of Texas-Houston in conjunction with the MD Anderson Cancer Center. While these groups do not offer referral services to practitioners in your area, they are useful to get a sense of what type of research is being conducted. You can even search for efforts specific to breast cancer should you decide to ask your own doctor about anything that piques your interest to learn more.

- **American Holistic Health Association**

    P.O. Box 17400
    Anaheim, CA 92817
    Phone: 714-779-6152
    Web site: www.ahha.org

    AHHA is "the leading national resource connecting people with vital solutions to reach a higher level of wellness." It provides free information to the public, including newsletters and referral lists of members located in your area. While it does not indicate practitioners who specialize in breast cancer, with board members like Deepak Chopra and Bernie Siegel, it's a reputable place to start.

    And of course, in addition to books and organizations, there are new Web sites appearing almost daily on this topic, from grassroots start-ups to "Yahoo Health: Alternative Medicine" as part of the Yahoo Internet search engine. Happy surfing. . . .

Rules of the Road for Family, Friends, and Other Participants

So finally you want to say, "Phew, we've gotten through this, so let's celebrate and get back to life." Not so fast. The completion of treatment and return to "normal" life can be a strange experience, one that is often isolating and lonely. The world expects her to be so happy that she's survived cancer that nothing else matters. Actually after surviving cancer, a lot of things—different things—matter. She'll be reassessing her life and what she wants out of it. So how can you help her through what might be an awkward time? How can you help her manage the transition from "patient" to "survivor"? And what kind of support might she need in her posttreatment "follow-up" days?

- **Don't slam the door shut. It's really not over yet.** Don't wipe out all the support and encouragement you've shown so far by just abruptly closing the door on the experience the minute treatment ends. Yes, you're at the end of the road, but you haven't arrived yet. Remember that she may go though a strange emotional roller coaster once treatment ends, and may need you along at her side for just a bit longer. Don't desert her now.

- **Calibrate the celebration sentiments.** Before you plan the victory party, calibrate her capacity to celebrate. She may be ready to declare victory in a big way, or may need some easing into the transition and would prefer reestablishing herself and her relationships in a more private way.

- **Plan a vacation.** Be a hero, and plan a vacation that will make her feel good, both body and soul. But ask her what she wants. She's had enough surprises over the past several months.

- **Think about how you ask, "How are you?"** Since she will regard these three little words as a very loaded question for quite a while to come, use this expression carefully and be sure of what you really mean by it. If you really want to know what she's thinking or feeling, you might ask the prolonged, "How *are* you?" and remain silent at the other end of the question to let her collect her thoughts and determine how she wants to address it. And be ready for the response.

- **Refer to her as a survivor.** Transform the conversation into the past tense. Refer to her as a survivor, and discuss "When you *had* breast cancer . . ." Watch her smile!

- **Remember who she was before breast cancer.** Begin to remember all those wonderful things about what she was "before BC" and begin to inquire about them again. It will surely be a lot more interesting to discuss a hobby of hers, an issue at work, or a community program in which she's involved, than whether her white blood counts were high enough to get her next round of chemotherapy. Remember her wit, her humor, her compassion, anything but her cancer.

- **Be a diligent companion for follow-up appointments.** Don't assume that just because she's done with treatments that she's also done with doctors' appointments. Offer to accompany her whenever she needs it. Many women feel entitled, given the crisis at hand, to burden people and ask them to disrupt their schedules during treatment. However, once it's past, many women are much more timid and awkward about asking for help, as they feel they've already burdened their support network enough. Help her avoid the awkwardness. Offer first.

- **Have a frank discussion about genetic testing.** If you are part of her immediate family, at some point it makes sense to have the discussion about whether she should go through genetic testing to determine whether other women in the family are at higher risk. However, the decision as to whether breast cancer should become a family affair is wrought with emotion, guilt, and fear, so tread lightly. You don't need to do it today, but sometime in the next year or so, when the situation is appropriate. However, don't even raise the subject unless the other women in the family are prepared to act on positive results, for example, enrollment in an early detection and prevention program.

- **Bring her news.** Although any woman who has been through the breast cancer experience will probably be wise enough to keep herself informed of major breakthroughs in treatment in case she should ever face a recurrence, she can't stay on top of it all. So, if you see something you think she may have missed, call it to her attention. She'll appreciate it.

Some Parting Thoughts

A Word on Staying Informed. Keep the Door Open, Just in Case.

Now that your entire ordeal has drawn to a conclusion, at least for now, you might feel that you just want to put this all behind you and get on with your life. You've been immersed in the cancer world long enough, living with it up close and personal. Yes, it is time to close the door and move on, but don't slam it shut. Keep it ajar just a tiny bit. In the unfortunate event you need to face a recurrence, you'll at least have the peace of mind that you're on top of the latest treatments. And if you don't, consider the basic knowledge your insurance policy.

Don't become obsessed with information gathering, but at the very minimum, you might monitor the newest breakthroughs and treatments a couple times a year. It's easy to do by simply following the media coverage of health and medical issues. Look at all the media hype in the past year or so over tamoxifen as a preventative for high-risk women. Alternatively, join one of the breast cancer associations like NABCO, The Breast Cancer Fund, or The Breast Cancer Coalition, and get their newsletters, or make it a habit to review breast cancer sites on the Internet a few times a year to see what's new. Some women even continue to meet with their support groups on an informal but regular basis, long after the group has officially disbanded. However, regardless of what information you find, as always, ask your health care team to put it in the context of what it means for you.

The Horizon Is No Longer Far Away in the Distant Skyline. It's Here.

Since we are the women who sit here having faced breast cancer, it may sound trite and irrelevant to say that major breakthroughs in the treatment and eradication of breast cancer are just over the horizon. To me, horizons have always evoked the image of an ever-shifting, unreachable, intangible destination far off in a distant landscape, somewhere you never reach no matter how hard you try to get there. Rethink that picture, please. Breast cancer breakthroughs are by and large here today. We can touch them, document them, and even envision what life will be like when we move beyond that horizon. Upon initial diagnosis, we all asked ourselves, "Why me?," and we all continue to yearn for an ever-elusive answer that we will never find.

In fact, our answer may simply be that there's never been a better time in the history of medical science to be fighting and conquering this disease. According to Dr. Larry Norton, Chief of Solid Tumor Medicine at Memorial Sloan-Kettering Cancer Center:

Even a casual student of contemporary science and medicine must appreciate that we are well into a renaissance in cancer medicine, the likes of which we have never seen before. The bases of life are molecules like DNA, and cancer is now known to be the result of abnormalities in these molecules. Our understanding of these molecules and our ability to intervene in their abnormalities has already led to significant advances and promises to lead rapidly toward the eradication of this disease. Right now we cure most cases of breast cancer, and every week brings advances that will enable us to cure more. We even have important leads regarding breast cancer prevention. Do I know the date on which cancer will be eliminated? Of course I do not. But I have every reason to be optimistic that a little girl born today will have little to fear from breast cancer forty or fifty years from now.

A NOTE FROM ALL THE DOCTORS

℞ *A Glimpse Over the Horizon: Promising Treatments on the Breast Cancer Front*

It would require another entire book to fully document all the exciting therapies and drugs in development today, a book that may be obsolete by the time it got to print, since advancements are accelerating so rapidly. Some very exciting new drugs and procedures are already approved for patient use, while others are under investigation in clinical trials.

Some of the advances of the past few years that are now available include:

- **Sentinel node biopsy.** No longer does every woman need to have her lymph nodes surgically removed by an axillary node dissection to determine if the cancer has spread beyond her breast into her body. Depending on the situation, she might be a candidate for the sentinel node biopsy, which will spare her the lifelong risks of lymph-edema and cellulitis. (See Chapter 5, "Long-Term Implications" for more.)
- **Cryoablation.** Early work of freezing tumors of very small size (essentially turning them into an ice ball with a probe placed in the tumor) and not surgically removing the lump is being investigated. In the future, this might be widely used or expanded to larger tumor size.
- **Redoing the lumpectomy.** In the past when lumpectomy and radiation therapy failed, mastectomy was the only recommended rescue treatment. Now in select situations, especially when a long interval exists between the first treatment and recurrence, recommendations might be made for re-excision (lumpectomy) and even localized radiation therapy.
- **Partial Breast Irradiation (PBI).** Radiation has traditionally been given to the entire breast after lumpectomy. There is growing enthusiasm for PBI either in the operating room at the time of lumpectomy or postoperatively via external radiation or internal devices placed

244 Some Parting Thoughts

within the lumpectomy site. This requires very select patients and circumstances.

- **Herceptin.** Herceptin is an antibody that targets HER2-neu, a protein on the surface of the cells of certain breast cancers. It is presently available for women who are "HER2-neu positive."
- **New applications for tamoxifen.** The proven use of tamoxifen to prevent breast cancer in susceptible women at high-risk, or "reinvention" from treatment to preventative, must be hailed as a breakthrough.
- **New drugs.** There are too many new drugs for breast cancer both on the market for patients with metastatic disease, and in clinical trials, to list. All drugs begin in the setting of metastatic disease (Taxol and Herceptin are excellent examples). Many make their way to the adjuvant setting (that's you!—somebody who does not have disease outside the breast and armpit) in time. So the treatment of patients with breast cancer just keeps getting better and better.

Other treatments that are on the horizon, under study but not yet commercially available, include:

- **Modulating resistance.** Theoretically, everyone who dies of breast cancer must have become resistant to chemotherapy. Therefore, if a way can be found to inhibit the ability of the cell to become resistant, then women can continue to receive chemotherapy to prolong their lives. Cancer cells may have a form of resistance called the multidrug resistance protein (MDR), which acts as a pump to shoot chemotherapy out of the cell before it can do its damage. Introducing a modulating resistance drug into the body to block MDR would enable the chemotherapy to accumulate in a cell to a level that results in cell death, the ultimate purpose of chemotherapy.
- **Tumor vaccines.** This promising science is in its infancy, but in some cases "immunizing" a patient against her own tumor can be an effective form of treatment, thereby preventing the cancer cells from damaging healthy tissues and organs. There is already a vaccine commercially

available for patients with prostate cancer called Provenge, made by the Dendreon Corporation.

- **Gene therapy.** What may come from the world-famous genome project remains an exciting unknown in cancer therapy. We may soon be able to predict how patients will tolerate a given chemotherapy drug by looking at gene expression of the enzymes responsible for breaking down the drugs. In effect, we may be able to develop "designer drugs" customized for how the chemical will interact with your own body's chemistry based on your genetic makeup.

And When It's All Over, Make a Contribution. Unfortunately, It Will Probably Help Someone You Love.

By the time you are through the entire breast cancer ordeal, you are probably exhausted, physically, emotionally, and especially financially. You probably feel like you have given 80 percent of your life savings to your doctors and hospitals. (But why not, because your only alternative was the risk of not having a life to save for?) Just do one more thing. Make a contribution that will help breast cancer in some way, shape, or form. It might be to the National Cancer Institute to fund research for a cure. It might be to the hospital where you were treated to support clinical trials at that institution or your own doctor's research. Or it might be to a local support group organization to help women who can't afford private counseling or care.

And it doesn't even have to be money. It might be your volunteer time or advocacy efforts. Volunteer to lead a local breast cancer support group. Sign up for a Komen Foundation "Race for the Cure." Or even consider participating in The Breast Cancer Fund's "Climb Against the Odds" mountain climb. In addition to this year's "Climb Against the Odds," my contribution has been writing this book with a twofold purpose: (1) hopefully to make life a bit easier for all those women who have yet to be faced with the challenge of beating breast cancer, and (2) to use some of the financial proceeds of this book to fund breast cancer research.

Make the donation in honor of all those friends, family, and even your doctors who have helped you get through this past year. Show your appreciation for all they have done. And with one in eight women facing breast cancer during their life, unfortunately you will probably also be helping someone else whom you know and love. Consider it insurance as well, because you might also be helping yourself, should you ever have to face a recurrence. But if we all work fast and furiously enough, someday we might just be able to say that our efforts did not just help one individual woman beat breast cancer, but that we actually triumphed over the disease, that we eradicated breast cancer out of our lives. Wouldn't that be nice?

And a Few Very Last Words . . .

Exactly one year, one month, and one day after my surgery, I stood atop a glacier near Mt. McKinley in Denali National Park, Alaska. After three days of mountain biking and then learning ice-climbing skills, I was amazed and awed that I was alive to be there, a bit wiser, a bit more reflective. I felt as strong, and as healthy, and as good as I ever had in my life. I felt on top of the world . . . literally. Who says breast cancer won't change you? It will. (I wouldn't have been so stupid to climb up a glacier before!) You, too, will get through your very own breast cancer experience. And survive with a smile. I wish you the best of luck.

Index